P9-BZT-277

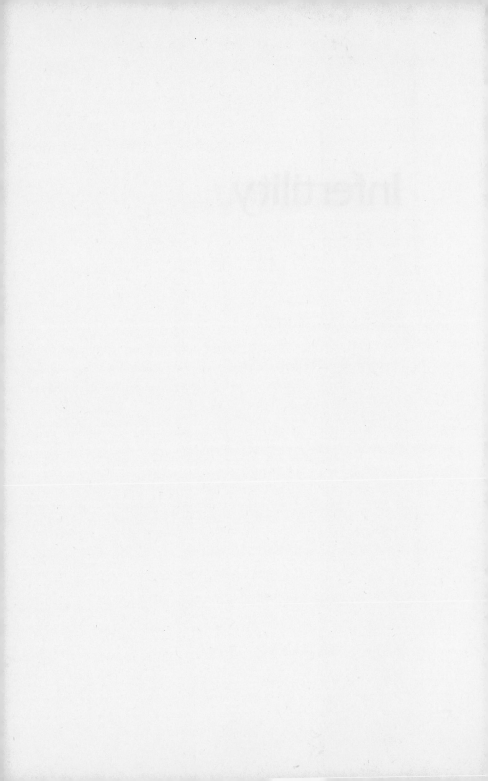

Infertility

Infertility

A COUPLE'S GUIDE TO
CAUSES AND TREATMENTS

Mary Harrison

Illustrations by William McCord

Houghton Mifflin Company Boston

1977

Copyright © 1977 by Mary Harrison

All rights reserved. No part of this work may be
reproduced or transmitted in any form by any means,
electronic or mechanical, including photocopying
and recording, or by any information storage
or retrieval system, without permission
in writing from the publisher.

Library of Congress Cataloging in Publication Data
Harrison, Mary.
   Infertility: a couple's guide to its causes and
treatments.
      Bibliography: p.   Includes index.
      1. Sterility.   I. Title.   [DNLM: 1. Sterility,
Female—Popular works.   2. Sterility, Male—Popular
works.   WP570 H321i]
RC889.H32   618.1'78   77-23506
ISBN 0-395-25375-6

Printed in the United States of America

V 10 9 8 7 6 5 4 3 2 1

This book is dedicated
to infertile people everywhere
and to the doctors who are
working to find solutions.

Author's Note

Six illustrations are grouped together following page 170. A glossary of medical terms begins on page 189. These will help the reader to understand unfamiliar or difficult terminology and procedures.

Contents

Illustrations

(following page 170)

Infertility

Learning from Experience

THE SCENE seems clear to me, even several years later — a cold room, green tiles, brilliant lights, and many masked faces asking me to put this arm here, that leg there. I tried to rest my cheeks on my hands, but the needles and IV tubes got in the way. How could I maintain this impossible position? My knees were under my chest, my hips in the air. I was sure the spinal anesthesia had not taken. I had felt the needle, and then the culdoscope, puncturing the wall of my vagina to enter the space on the other side. The anesthesiologist kept telling the Harvard medical student, as if in apology, that I was tall, that sometimes with tall girls the spinal anesthesia was not so deep as it could be. The discomfort was minor, however, compared to my curiosity. Someone was actually looking inside me, at my ovaries, my fallopian tubes.

I tried hard to hear the masked voice at the foot of the operating table. "Encapsulated right ovary." A pause. "Kinking of the right tube." Another pause. And then, "Endometrial adhesions, endometriosis around the left ovary."

"Endometriosis?" I asked, and without waiting for the answer, "Now someone will believe me. I *told* them I had endometriosis, but no one thought I did. I knew I did, I told them . . ." The words spilled out, undoubtedly loosened by the medication; I could not stop them. I was relieved that something was in fact wrong, exultant to have *my* diagnosis confirmed, and, then, angry that it had taken so many years to discover.

The culdoscope was removed, people began to untangle my arms and legs. Once more on my back, I finally saw the doctor's face, but my questions received only a laconic "Yes, it can be treated."

As they transferred me from the operating table, the medical student, a young girl with intense dark eyes, leaned over me and asked, "How did you know you had endometriosis?"

"I couldn't get pregnant," I answered. "And I had changes in menstrual pain which none of the doctors thought were serious."

"Oh," she murmured, "these male doctors, they've never even *had* a period!"

And they wheeled me out to the recovery room.

It had taken three and a half years to discover the cause of my infertility. In that time, I had consulted five gynecologists, two psychiatrists, and a divorce lawyer. One of the doctors had told me all was well, to relax and forget about it. Another had told me that there was possibly a problem with the fallopian tubes, but he had warned me that operations on the tubes generally did not succeed. Still another had attributed the infertility solely to a male factor, a borderline low sperm count. One of the psychiatrists, a woman, had urged me not to leave therapy, implying that my infertility was psychosomatic, a diagnosis she made before many important tests had been performed. And a solicitous but naive friend had cited a health food addict's admonition to eat some special food to "cure" infertility.

In the course of those three and a half years, my husband and I had heard many conflicting opinions. I had received incomplete workups. And together we had been hesitant about pushing ahead.

What took us so long? With two doctorate degrees we should have known better. But my husband had received his training in gynecology years before and only as part of the medical school curriculum, and my field was far from medicine. We were also human. We thought everything was possible. We had planned our life so that schooling and training came first, and then children. We fully believed that the first shot at conception would result in pregnancy. We simply could not believe it when we failed to conceive after the first two months of trying. People began to ask us when we were going to start a family. "Soon," we replied nervously. Everyone else seemed to get pregnant with ease. In fact, most people seemed to be avoiding *another* pregnancy. So we accepted the first diagnoses that the sperm count was within normal limits and that my pelvic anatomy was fine. "Just be patient," the doctors told us. We started to wait, never considering turning to an infertility specialist at that time. Humanly — and desperately — we wanted to be normal.

However, after the first few months went by with no results, my scholar's training and curiosity led me first to my husband's gynecology texts and then to a medical library. My earliest research threw me directly into a sea of differing opinions and theories. The study of infertility seemed hardly an exact science. There did seem to be general agreement, however, about what tests the basic infertility workup should include. I began to consider asking my doctor for some of those tests. And naively, I made my own diagnosis, which was confirmed — to everyone's surprise — several years later.

In retrospect I am startled at the way we felt when our quest began. Even though we were the ones who decided to initiate the workup, we still felt ambivalent. I knew that my reaction to one of the tests was in no way similar to the reaction described in the textbooks, but I found it difficult to contradict the doctor's positive reading of the test. After all, he was a respected obstetrician-gynecologist, even though he was not a specialist in infertility. My husband and I simply kept hoping I would get pregnant. We clung to every positive sign, even when reason suggested otherwise. We were pulled along on a will to believe until we became the two sides in a tug-of-war, with the urologist adamantly insisting that my husband was fine and the first of my gynecologists insisting equally adamantly that I was fine. Our marriage began to tear apart, though neither of us was willing to admit that the infertility had anything to do with it. It was difficult even to admit we were an infertile couple.

Only when we began to talk about our problem with another couple who had been through a similar situation did we begin to assess our problem more rationally. Our friends had been told they were "normal" when, in fact, there were serious but curable problems. They had sought the help of specialists and now had two children. Perhaps there was hope for us.

There was indeed hope for us, but it was a long time coming. Knowledge was essential. We both knew more questions had to be asked and answered. What would have happened if we had accepted the first diagnosis? How many childless couples have accepted a similar erroneous first diagnosis? Clearly hindsight is better than foresight. We only hope our hindsight can help other couples in the same dilemma.

This book is the product of my experience as a patient, and it is intended as a patient's guide to infertility. It is not a medical textbook, but you will find references to medical works that can be consulted for further information. The book will introduce you to the extreme complexity of the problem of infertility, and it will tell you something about dealing with the problem. The first section presents the complexities of normal conception so that you can understand more clearly the innumerable areas where problems can arise. You will discover how many aspects of normal conception remain a mystery and will be able to appreciate more fully the enigmas that still remain in the field of infertility. The next few sections address the questions that arise as you start to deal with your own problem. How do you decide you have a problem? Where do you go for help? What tests should be performed to guarantee a complete and thorough evaluation? What treatments are available for various problems? What hope do they promise? The final sections present related problems, such as habitual miscarriage and secondary infertility, and they also raise some questions about the future of infertility. Throughout the book you will accompany me on the research I began when I discovered I had the problem.

Going beyond mere description and enumeration of tests and treatments, however, the book is also a sort of personal journal of the fears and doubts, anxieties and heartaches that are part of the problem of infertility. Our own experiences will weave through the book not only to demonstrate the pitfalls of an infertility investigation but also, and perhaps more important, to let you know you are not alone, to share with you the painful emotional journey we all go through in infertility.

The book is rooted in my own mistakes and based on my firm belief that knowledge of a problem makes you a better patient. Years ago, I had to investigate the problem for myself surreptitiously in a medical library. But the knowledge I gained started me on the right road. I found out that I could read my own body, that I was the best one to note the slight changes in my own particular patterns of normal. I realized that I could understand the tests recommended in infertility textbooks. I gained the confidence that I could and should ask for tests that had not been performed up to that time.

You can too. Learn what we had to learn. Profit from our mistakes. With fewer babies available for adoption, it is crucial that all couples who want to have children and cannot conceive at will, receive the most thorough examination possible. With many questions about the causes and treatments of infertility still unanswered, it is crucial that all infertile couples have the benefit of the knowledge which medical science does have about the problem. Advances have been made in the past few years and solutions have been found for many problems. Experiments are going on that promise new hope. What seemed a hopeless situation in our grandmothers' days is not so hopeless today.

PART ONE

The Nature
of the Problem

CHAPTER I

What Is Infertility?

INFERTILITY IS involuntary childlessness. A couple wants to have a child and cannot conceive in spite of all their efforts. This does not mean that their problem is simply not achieving a pregnancy the first time they try. According to the standard medical definition, they will be diagnosed as infertile when the woman does not become pregnant after a year of intercourse without contraception. One full year! Twelve months of trying — and not succeeding. Twelve menstrual periods that come so regularly that they are literally a "curse," a constant reminder of failure. Making love loses its joy. And no one seems to understand.

The many myths and misunderstandings about infertility only compound your problem. Those who take fertility for granted are often misguided in the advice they give so freely, as was my friend who urged me to eat wheat germ. Those who suffer from infertility may have mistaken ideas that prevent them from obtaining proper treatment.

So at the outset it is important to clear up the misunderstandings, to define terms, to state clearly and explicitly what infertility is — and what it is not.

Infertility is not *a rare condition.* When you discover your infertility, you feel alone. Newspapers and television constantly remind you of the problems of overpopulation. Your friends seem either to be pregnant or to be avoiding another pregnancy. Your problem seems unique to you. It is not.

Over five million couples in the English-speaking world share your problem. Three and a half million of them are in the United States and Canada alone. One in ten couples wants to have a first child and cannot.[1] Three in twenty couples want to have a second or third child and cannot.[2]

Infertility is not *just a "woman's disease."* The popular notion that the woman is always the barren partner is deeply imbedded in the western world. The Judaeo-Christian tradition abounds with barren women — Sarah, Rebecca, Rachel, St. Anne, to name only a few. In more recent history, rulers have given up their wives if they did not become pregnant. Even today, in most cases of infertility, it is the woman who seeks help first. But the condition is not confined to women.

Infertility is a couple's problem. Two individual systems must each be working correctly before they can work together successfully to create a child. When pregnancy does not occur, both partners must be evaluated.

Doctors estimate that a male problem exists in 30 to 40 percent of all infertility cases, a female problem in 60 to 70 percent.[3] Some specialists estimate that, in a large percentage of cases, more than one problem is at work causing the infertility.[4] It is thus imperative that all systems in both partners be tested completely and thoroughly.

Infertility is not *confined to one particular group.* Any person of childbearing age can encounter the problem. An infertile person can come from any social or economic class, from any race or religion. There is no distinct profile of the infertile person. If puberty has been normal and if there are no impediments to normal intercourse, you have little way of knowing in advance if you will have a problem with infertility.

Infertility can *happen to people who have been fertile earlier in their lives.* Why? Fertility is not constant from puberty on. It is obvious that fertility can be dramatically curtailed by serious injury to any of the genital organs. But beyond that, fertility can also be adversely affected by diseases and, important for women, by age.

Even though a fertile man is likely to remain so most of his life, certain conditions may threaten his fertility. He can have inflammation of the testicles, orchitis, caused by mumps, which can permanently affect his fertility. He can be overexposed to radiation. Even if he does not encounter these drastic situations, a normal man may find that his fertility varies considerably during his adult life, influenced by fatigue, fever, or stress. His fertility can also be affected by some drugs and medications or overexposure of the testicles to heat. Most of these variations in fertility are usually temporary, but you should know that they can sometimes occur.

A normal woman's fertility, on the other hand, has a much shorter life span. We all know that a normal woman is fertile only from puberty until menopause. But like the male, she too can encounter problems which will impair her fertility. Infertility in a woman may occur as a result of certain diseases, such as gonorrhea and other pelvic infections. Endometriosis and fibroid tumors can also affect fertility, and these conditions seem more likely to occur as a woman grows older. Sometimes infertility can even be related to problems that arise after a normal pregnancy.

Most important, a woman's fertility is affected by age, decreasing steadily from age thirty on. One authoritative study has shown that one in ten previously fertile women will be infertile by age thirty-five, one in three by age forty, and seven in eight by age forty-five.[5] A woman's fertility ends when menopause is over.

Too many people think infertility is "all in your head." Unfortunately, this "diagnosis" seems to have great popularity with the general public. Some fertile people who are doing their best to avoid pregnancy find it hard to believe that anyone has difficulty becoming pregnant. So they offer their ill-founded advice, "It must be all in your head." I heard it from a physician and from a relative who is not a physician, and women I know have heard it from their best friends, and even from their mothers.

When I heard it from a physician, the effect was devastating. My investigation had hardly begun when a psychiatrist, instead of advising me to continue all the tests, suggested my infertility might be psychosomatic.

The diagnosis of psychosomatic infertility should not be made until all systems have been thoroughly checked and all the tests have been performed, and until the doctor has good evidence that psychological problems are at work. There are, in fact, some psychological problems that do impair a couple's fertility, but they can often be clearly defined. Sexual problems, such as impotence or severe frigidity, may prevent normal intercourse. Sometimes psychological factors may disrupt the functioning of the endrocrine system and thereby affect fertility.

When a specific cause for infertility cannot be found, this does not mean that the cause has to be psychological. Many physicians feel it is more correct to cite the limits of knowledge than to cite the psychological causes for all cases of unexplained infertility. As a patient, I would agree. First, this answer seems more honest. Second, after all tests have been made, it would seem easier for a patient to accept the conclusion that the physicians simply do not know the cause than to spend the rest of your life wondering what is wrong with your psyche that prevents you from having a child.

There is no such medical entity as a "normal" infertile couple. In the past doctors have used this term to describe the couple in whom no cause of infertility can be found. However, this failure of diagnosis does not mean that unexplained infertility is a normal state. If a couple want to have a child and are unable to, something is wrong. Before the discovery of immunological causes of infertility, many couples with that problem must have been told that their infertility could not be explained. If the medical profession cannot find a cause, it is only an indication of the limits of knowledge. It does not mean that the couple is "normal."

Infertility is not *always an irreversible condition,* although it was considered so in the past. It was proof of their faith that barren women of the Bible finally did bear children, a divine cure to an otherwise hopeless state. Today a majority of the recognized problems that cause infertility can be treated. The success rates measured in terms of subsequent pregnancy vary, but advances in treatment methods have been made and continue to be made. Forty years ago, only 10 percent of infertile couples could be helped to achieve a pregnancy. Today some experts estimate that 40 to 50 percent of them can be helped to have a child.[6] Tomorrow perhaps even a larger percentage will be able to become parents.

CHAPTER 2

The Complexity of Normal Conception *

OUR FERTILITY is something we all take for granted, until we find out otherwise. In fact, most of the lay books on pregnancy and fetal development start with the assumption that complexities begin *after* conception has occurred, after the two germ cells, sperm and ovum, have met and begun the process of development into a human being. Yet, for five million couples in the English-speaking world, getting pregnant seems far more problematic.

"But all it takes is one sperm and one egg," countless infertile couples have often said in frustration. They are right, but the road leading up to that union is long and rutted with pitfalls. Indeed, considering all the systems that must be working correctly and all the events that must happen at exactly the right time, it is a wonder that so many conceptions do occur. In order to understand the multiple causes of infertility, it is absolutely essential to understand the intricacies of normal conception.

The male starts preparations early, some estimate as long as two and a half months before the event.[1] It takes that long to

---

* The reader is referred to Figures 1–4, following page 170, for diagrams of Conception, Female Genital Organs, Male Genital Organs, and Glands Involved in Reproduction in the Male and in the Female.

produce a mature spermatozoon, a microscopic cell only $1/6000$ of an inch in diameter and $1/500$ of an inch in length.

Spermatogenesis, the production of mature sperm, takes place in the mature descended male testicles, but the process is still only poorly understood. It depends on an involved network of relationships between part of the brain and four different glands. These are: the hypothalamus, an area of the brain considered by most authorities as the master control of the glands; the pituitary gland, located next to the hypothalamus; the thyroid gland, located in the neck; the adrenal glands, located near the kidneys; and the testicles, or testes, located in the scrotum. These four glands secrete several different hormones which circulate in the blood and influence, directly and indirectly, the production of mature sperm. These hormones are: interstitial cell-stimulating hormone (ICSH) and follicle-stimulating hormone (FSH), produced by the pituitary; thyroxin, produced by the thyroid; cortisone and small amounts of the sexual hormones, androgen and estrogen, produced by the adrenal glands; and testosterone, produced by the testicles. A correct balance among all these hormones is absolutely necessary to produce mature sperm. Underproduction or overproduction of any one hormone can throw the system off and affect fertility. For example, even though the thyroid gland is not directly responsible for the creation of sperm, it can cause infertility. The function of thyroxin in the body is to control the speed at which the organs work. If the thyroid produces too much or too little thyroxin, it will interfere with the normal rate at which the other glands function and thus affect fertility.

The two hormones that are most directly involved in the creation of sperm are FSH and ICSH, secreted by the pituitary. FSH, which takes its name from the similar hormone that stimulates the growth of follicles in the ovaries of women, stimulates the production of sperm in the seminiferous tubules in the testicles. ICSH stimulates the production of testosterone in the interstitial cells in the testicles. Testosterone is necessary for the production of sperm; it also stimulates other glands in the male

genital tract to produce the liquid that carries the sperm out of
the testicles through the urethra in an ejaculation.

Sperm do not come into being in one single act, but rather
each sperm is the result of several complicated cell divisions.
At any one time, millions of these divisions are going on in the
seminiferous tubules to produce the millions of sperm which are
found in each ejaculate. Although only one sperm cell will
eventually meet and mate with the egg, one hundred to two
hundred *million* sperm are the optimal number in each ejaculation to assure fertility. This may seem an enormous number,
but, even so, the supply of sperm is not exhausted after one
ejaculation. Within thirty-six to forty-eight hours, or even
sooner according to some estimates, another adequate supply of
mature sperm is ready. From puberty to death, males continuously produce millions of sperm; they are always prepared for
any eventuality. Every time a male ejaculates a normal amount
of normal sperm, he is potentially fertile.

The situation is different with the female. From puberty
to menopause, a woman usually produces only one mature
egg or ovum each month, preparing herself not just for any
eventuality but for one special encounter. In contrast to the
male, she is not potentially fertile every time she has intercourse. In contrast to the male, she does not continuously gen-
erate egg cells throughout her life, but rather is born with a
given supply of eggs. During the woman's fertile lifetime some
of these eggs will grow to maturity, but the majority will never
even ripen for possible fertilization. Nevertheless a woman's
body recurrently prepares itself for pregnancy. Between puberty and menopause, each time an egg is not fertilized and
menstruation occurs, her body immediately begins again to produce another egg.

It takes a few weeks for a mature egg to ripen. It is the larg-
est single human cell, although only $1/200$ of an inch in diameter. The maturational process of an egg, like that of the sperm,
depends on a similar series of interactions among the glands.
These interactions are better understood in the female, and treat-

ments have been found for many of the malfunctions of the glands. You should understand how the glandular systems work to insure female fertility.

In the female, the hypothalamus is involved along with four glands — the pituitary, the thyroid, the adrenals, and the ovaries. The glands produce some of the same hormones that are at work in male fertility, but other hormones are also secreted. The pituitary produces follicle-stimulating hormone (FSH) and luteinizing hormone (LH), which is the same hormone as ICSH in the male. The thyroid produces thyroxin. Androgen and cortisone are produced by the adrenals, and estrogen and progesterone by the ovaries.

In the female, as in the male, the area of the brain known as the hypothalamus is apparently the master control of the glandular system, stimulating the pituitary to produce hormones. But this is not its only function. Because the hypothalamus is a key center of the entire central nervous system, it also serves as a kind of "clearing house of various positive and negative impulses gathered from the body's internal and external environments." [2] Because of this larger role, researchers feel that the hypothalamus is probably the route by which anxieties and stresses registered in the brain affect the functioning of the pituitary and possibly of the other glands.

In the female, as in the male, the thyroid and adrenal glands are also involved in the reproductive process. Underactivity or overactivity of these glands can adversely affect the reproductive process.

The most basic of the glandular interactions involved in producing an egg will be described here. First, FSH produced by the pituitary passes into the blood stream and focuses on one of several follicles or egg sacs in the ovary to cause growth. Second, as the follicle begins to mature it puts out the hormone estrogen, which, as one of its many functions, causes a thickening of the lining of the uterus, the endometrium. Third, the increased estrogen, as another of its functions, stimulates the pituitary gland to cut down its production of FSH and to increase its production of LH, which focuses on the same ovarian follicle and causes the mature egg to be released. It is finally free to be fertilized, but the hormonal process goes on. Fourth, the now empty follicle turns a bright yellow-orange, at which point it takes the name *corpus luteum* (Latin for "yellow body"), and it produces progesterone and estrogen, which results in a further thickening of the uterine lining, preparing it to receive the fertilized egg. If the egg is fertilized, it travels through the fallopian tube to the uterus to implant in the uterine lining. If implantation occurs, the corpus luteum continues, in the very early stages of pregnancy, to produce estrogen and progesterone to maintain and enrich that lining. However, if the egg is not fertilized, the egg disintegrates, the corpus luteum begins to break up, and there is a sharp drop in the production of estrogen and progesterone, all of this followed by menstruation, in which the lining of the uterus is passed out through the cervix and the vagina.

The most crucial moment for conception occurs at the third step. A mature egg, released from the ovary, is now a free agent, ready to be fertilized. What next? Contrary to common belief, the egg is *not* automatically ejected directly into the fallopian tubes. The tubes that transport the egg are attached to the uterus at one end, but near the ovaries they hang free in the abdomen, the peritoneal cavity. The free end of the fallopian tube is made up of tissues resembling tentacles, called fimbriae. These fimbriae must find their way to the ovary, wrap themselves around the lower half, and seize the egg as it is extruded.[3] Apparently, the left tube must make contact with the left ovary and the right tube with the right ovary in order to capture the single egg, which is usually produced by only one of the ovaries each month. In very rare instances, one of the tubes may cross to the other ovary to capture the egg.[4] Once the tube has captured the egg, the egg begins its four- to five-day journey, waved along by small hairs or cilia in the tube toward the uterus.

For fertilization of this egg to take place, a supply of healthy spermatozoa must be deposited inside the vagina, near the mouth of the cervix. The sperm are all equipped with individual tails that enable them to propel themselves forward. Like salmon, they must swim upstream, first passing through the cervix, then navigating the relatively ample space of the uterus, then finding their way to the small openings of the tubes, only one of which leads to the single egg, and finally swimming against the currents of the hairs in the tube to reach the area of the tube where fertilization must take place.

Ideally one hundred to two hundred *million* sperm are deposited in the vagina, but only a small proportion of these arrive in the outer third of the correct tube. Only one of these will fertilize the egg. Why do so few arrive? Obviously, the journey is long, and sperm are lost at every stage. In addition, many sperm cannot swim and simply remain in the vagina. Those that do swim prefer an alkaline environment, and the more acid secretions of the vagina can inhibit their progress. If there is infection present, white blood cells can destroy sperm. If antibodies are present, they can immobilize sperm. Finally, once past the cervix (which produces more alkaline secretions at the time of ovulation), the distance to be covered is enormous. The environment is more welcoming, but the sperm must travel a distance of approximately three thousand times its own length. This is the equivalent of a person six feet tall swimming three miles upstream! But navigating an enormous distance is not the only challenge for the sperm. There is also the question of timing.

For fertilization to take place, the sperm must meet the egg in the outer third of the tube during the egg's fertile lifetime, an extraordinarily short period of from twelve to twenty-four hours. Since, according to some estimates, sperm can live only as long as forty-eight hours, they may arrive early and wait for the egg. But there is a period that probably lasts only twenty-four to forty-eight hours each month when fertilization can occur.

If fertilization does not occur, the egg begins to disintegrate and is eventually sloughed off. If, on the other hand, the sperm and egg meet, the complicated process of cell division leading to a new human life begins in the fallopian tube. The fertilized egg or blastocyst then moves toward the uterus over the next few days, undergoing changes which are still only poorly understood. By the end of four to five days, it comes to rest in the uterus, ready to undergo changes which will allow it to burrow into the lining already prepared for it by the action of the hormones put out by the ovaries. The embryo can then begin its development. Conception has taken place. What many people consider the easiest part has happened in its amazingly complex way.

CHAPTER 3

The Myriad Causes of Infertility

ALL OF THE EVENTS described in the preceding chapter go on naturally and normally in most of the adult population — so normally, in fact, that preventing conception has become a primary global concern. In spite of the number and complexity of the steps involved in the reproductive process, 80 to 85 percent of couples do not encounter any difficulties in achieving a pregnancy. But what of the other 15 to 20 percent of couples?

In a very small number of cases, certain congenital problems may seriously impede or totally prevent fertility. These include the absence or gross malformation of any part of the genital system in either male or female, and certain rare chromosomal abnormalities. These unusual conditions may be discovered at puberty when maturational problems arise. However, sometimes the absence or malformation of an organ or chromosomal disorders are only discovered in the course of an infertility investigation.

What other causes of infertility turn up in an investigation? In some cases the causes are blatant, and the solutions may be easy. Sometimes a couple is not having intercourse properly. The male may simply not be inserting his penis into his partner's vagina, and hence pregnancy is impossible. As extraordinary as this seems in our era of sexual openness, doctors have written that they do find an intact hymen or opening of the vagina in some of the women who come for an infertility workup. Doctors also find couples who consistently fail to have intercourse during the woman's fertile period.* In these two situations, education about sexual technique and the reproductive process may be the solutions for the problem. Infrequently, severe stress, extreme malnutrition, or poor general health can be responsible for infertility. The dramatically lowered birth rate during the siege of Leningrad in the Second World War is concrete evidence of this. The cessation of stress, improvements in general diet and health, may be the solution for these problems.

However, if these obvious causes are not at work, what else can turn up in the evaluation of infertility? A male condition is present in 30 to 40 percent of all infertility cases, a female condition in 60 to 70 percent of the cases. Yet, the statistics are far from clear, as the variations in percentages indicate. Diagnosis can be complicated by the fact that more than one problem may be at work causing the infertility. Indeed, authorities estimate that there are multiple causes in 35 to 80 percent of all infertility cases. Each partner may have a problem. One or both members of the pair may have several problems. There are also puzzling cases of infertility that seem to have no apparent cause. Some specialists find this in as many as 20 percent of their infertility cases. Others find it in only 5 to 10 percent.[1] All these varying statistics reveal much about the changing state of knowledge about infertility. They do not, however, shed much light on the specific causes of infertility.

The three general causes are very basic: faulty production of the germ cells, sperm and egg; impediments to the meeting of sperm and egg and subsequent fertilization; faulty implantation of the fertilized egg in the uterus. These causes are easy to un-

* The fertile period varies from woman to woman, but it usually occurs about fourteen days before the onset of menstruation. It is important to stress that this is *usually* the case, because there can be variations in the occurrence of the fertile period. Some of the tests described on pages 59–61, 69–71 can aid in establishing the approximate time of fertility.

derstand, but the mechanisms by which they operate are sometimes very complicated. There are any number of problems in the male — endocrinological, physical, and psychological — that can interfere with the production and transport of sperm, just as the same problems in the female can interfere with the production, fertilization, and implantation of the egg. Because the problems are so numerous, it would be impossible to mention every one of them in this chapter. This discussion will include only the most common causes of infertility in both male and female. The tests to uncover the causes and the treatments available for specific problems will be described later in the book.

Male Problems

In order to be fertile, a man must produce an adequate amount of normal sperm and must be able to deposit that sperm in a woman's vagina. The principal causes of infertility in the male, then, are faulty production of sperm and problems with depositing sperm in the wife's vagina.

Faulty production of sperm shelters a host of problems relating to the quantity, quality, and motility of sperm. Sperm may be absent or few in number. They may be abnormal in shape. They may be relatively sluggish or immobile. These problems are difficult because their causes are not fully understood. Indeed, physicians have been able to suggest only a few basic reasons for them. In some cases the cause may be endocrinological. The pituitary gland may not secrete enough of its hormones to stimulate the production of sperm in the testicles. The malfunction of other glands, such as the thyroid or adrenals, can also interfere with the production of sperm. The cause may be developmental. The testicles may not have descended into the scrotum, or they may have descended too late, after the male entered puberty. Certain diseases or abnormal conditions may be involved. Mumps orchitis in puberty or adulthood can prevent fertility. Varicocele, a dilation of testicular veins, also interferes with fertility, but recently this condition has been treated successfully with surgery. Environmental factors may interfere with spermatogenesis, but in many cases they impair fertility only temporarily. Among these factors are: poor nutrition; certain allergies; individual sensitivities to tobacco, alcohol, or marijuana; reactions to certain medications; or injury of the testicles. Excess heat around the testicles is also a culprit. The chief reason the testicles are outside the body in the scrotum is so that they can be cooler than the normal body temperature of 98.6 F degrees. When the temperature of the testicles is raised — by illness with a high fever, tight underwear, or even prolonged hot baths — the production of sperm can be impaired for a time.

Interference with the transport and depositing of sperm is probably more rarely encountered than problems with sperm production. The chief physical cause is one of actual barrier. The paths that the sperm travel within the testicle to the penis may be blocked, either because of disease or injury or because of congenital malformations, which are found in only 1 percent of infertile men.[2] Two very rare physical conditions, hypospadias and retrograde ejaculation, can interfere with the passage and depositing of sperm. (See pages 124–25.)

Other conditions interfering with the transport and depositing of sperm are impotence, premature ejaculation outside the vagina, and ejaculatory incompetence. In impotence the man is unable to have an erection and therefore cannot have intercourse. In premature ejaculation outside the vagina, the man is able to have an erection but he ejaculates his sperm before insertion. In ejaculatory incompetence, the man has an erection but cannot ejaculate.

A host of psychological problems may be at the root of these conditions. Anxiety, depression, and alcoholism are the most frequent psychological syndromes encountered. But you should know that impotence can be associated with certain diseases such as hypothyroidism or diabetes. It can also be a side effect of some drugs and certain medications such as tranquilizers, antidepressants, and preparations used in the treatment of high blood pressure.

Female Problems

In order to be fertile, a woman must produce a normal egg that can pass from the ovary into the fallopian tube. She must have an open pathway for sperm to travel from the vagina, through the cervix and uterus, into the fallopian tubes. And her uterus must be properly prepared and able to receive a fertilized egg.

Problems with the fallopian tubes occur in 20 to 35 percent of all cases of female infertility, problems with ovulation in 10 to 15 percent, problems with the cervix in 5 to 20 percent.[3] Other problems include malfunction of the thyroid or adrenal glands; infections or inflammations of the genital organs; and immunologic incompatibilities or allergies of the wife to the husband's sperm. Frigidity and vaginismus, a constriction of the vagina, can cause infertility if they prevent a woman from having intercourse.

Why should these problems arise? The answers are as complex as the reproductive system itself. Only the most basic theories will be suggested here. Problems with ovulation are usually, but not always, related to malfunction of the endocrinological system. The pituitary gland may not stimulate the ovaries, or the ovaries may fail to respond to the messages sent out by the pituitary. Malfunctioning of the thyroid or adrenal glands can also interfere with ovulation. Problems with the fallopian tubes are usually related to physical conditions. The fallopian tubes may be completely or partially blocked, or they may be unable to move as freely as they should. Blockages may be the result of either congenital malformations or diseases of the pelvis, such as gonorrhea. Relative immobility of the tubes may be caused by adhesions or scarring. Problems with the cervix include, but are not limited to, physical blockages such as growths or polyps, infections or inflammations, the production of "hostile" cervical mucus, and physical weakness of the cervical muscles. The failure of a fertilized egg to implant in the uterus may be the result of the production of an inadequate uterine lining. Finally, extreme frigidity and vaginismus are usually, but not always, related to psychological problems.

Habitual Miscarriage

Habitual miscarriage is another cause of infertility. A couple may have no difficulty conceiving, but the woman is consistently unable to carry the pregnancy to term. Miscarriage can occur in any woman and does occur in 10 percent of all pregnancies, usually as a result of defects in the egg or sperm or of faulty implantation in the uterus. In infertility, miscarriage is considered a significant factor when it occurs three times in a row. This constitutes habitual miscarriage.

What causes habitual miscarriage? The same disorders that can cause isolated miscarriage — defective germ cells and faulty implantation. Researchers have also offered other explanations, some of which are widely accepted, while others are the subject of great disagreement.[4] Like the causes of infertility itself, those suggested for habitual miscarriage fall into four categories: physical, endocrinological, immunological, and psychological.

The physical causes are clear-cut, though they may not be discovered until they have already resulted in one miscarriage. They include physical defects of the uterus, which can range from a congenitally abnormally shaped uterus to a weak cervix to growths within the uterus that interfere with the implantation of the egg or encourage uterine contraction.

Some of the endocrinological causes are also well understood, but there are arguments about whether these factors are primary. Early deficiencies in progesterone have been isolated as a reason for habitual early miscarriage occurring within a week or two of fertilization. Some researchers suspect that other hormonal imbalances may be responsible for miscarriages that occur later than the first few weeks of pregnancy.[5]

More speculative are the suggestions that immunologic reactions, psychological upsets, and dietary deficiencies are responsible for habitual miscarriage. (The arguments for and against these theories will be discussed in Chapter 15.)

Secondary Infertility

Fifteen percent of all married couples have one child and then find that they are unable to have another one. Congenital malformations of the genital organs and chromosomal abnormalities are usually not involved, because these would most likely have prevented the first pregnancy. But many of the factors involved in primary infertility can develop. For example, a male may develop a low sperm count because of disease, fatigue, stress, or injury. A female may develop problems with ovulation for similar reasons. Or a woman may develop physical problems with the genital organs, such as fibroid tumors, polyps, or endometriosis. Other problems in women may arise as a direct result of the first pregnancy. The cervix may have been damaged during the expulsion of the baby. Mild postpartum infection may have caused blockages in the fallopian tubes.

The Problem of Unexplained Infertility

In 5 to 20 percent of all infertility cases, doctors are not able to find the reason. In spite of all the knowledge that experts do have about infertility, they are still puzzled about many aspects of the reproductive process. If some of these puzzles are solved, doctors may uncover subtle factors responsible for those cases of infertility which seem to have no apparent cause. Some of the following questions are being asked.

What causes the fallopian tubes to move to the ovaries to pick up the egg?

What happens in the fallopian tubes to promote the meeting of the sperm and egg?

How does the sperm "find" the egg? Exactly how is the sperm prepared to enter and fertilize the egg?

What effect does the seminal fluid have on the sperm which it contains? Is there any way to improve it, if it is defective?

PART TWO

Infertility—
Your Problem

CHAPTER 4

When Do You Decide You Have a Problem?

THIS QUESTION may sound odd to people who have never experienced infertility. Those who get pregnant with ease may say, "Don't be silly. It's simple. You know you have a problem if you don't get pregnant. Subject closed." But the answer is not quite so simple. My husband and I know that from experience.

The summer of 1969 is unforgettable for us for two reasons. On July 20 of that year the Americans made the first successful landing on the moon. In the dark decade of the sixties it was at last good to be an American. In Rome we gasped in amazement, joined the crowds of Italians cheering Armstrong and Aldrin, and forgot the scorching heat that beat against the red walls of the city. That night, with all the windows open, we made the first of many unsuccessful attempts to have a baby. We anticipated no problems, and we laughed as we thought how lucky our child would be to be conceived in Rome — and on the night of the first moon walk. The moon landing was an immediately resounding success; the baby making was a fizzle.

But we found any number of ways to rationalize our situation as the summer dragged into fall, and vacation turned back into work. My husband remembered how the heat of Rome had driven us both to take cold baths at one in the morning.

"That must be it," he said. "You never should have taken

that bath." As a physician he knew that baths were not effective contraceptives. If they were, the population problem would not exist. But emotionally he needed an explanation for our failure.

I found other ways to explain our lack of success in July. And then in August. And again in September. In August it was, "We must have missed the right day this month. We'll try again next month." In September, "I guess I got up too soon after making love." In October, "Maybe my Ph.D. exams are getting me so upset that I am not ovulating." Inwardly, I doubted these explanations, but each was some kind of cause that would be only temporary. At least I hoped so. I was, in fact, anxious — over the upcoming exams, over this failure of my body, over the problem of infertility that neither of us was willing to call by name.

"Why did I ever think of trying to get pregnant," I groaned, "with my exams coming up?" Sleepless nights, the first signs of gray hair, and increasing self-doubts. I lost confidence in everything. How could I pass the exams, if I couldn't even get pregnant? What kind of woman was I?

I was due for a regular gynecological checkup in October. I had made the appointment months before, thinking that it would be my first prenatal visit. How wrong I had been! Everything seemed normal in the checkup. And when the doctor heard we'd been trying to conceive for only a few months, he contributed to our rationalizing by saying that there was no reason to begin worrying — at least not yet.

"You're twenty-nine?" he asked, checking my records. I nodded assent — and for the first time began to get an inkling that age is a factor in infertility. For the first time I began to wonder if my pursuit of a career had closed the door to motherhood. But the doctor smiled comfortingly and told me to wait a few months and see what happened.

Later in the year, when it became increasingly obvious that something must be wrong, we found other ways to rationalize. We decided we must have "marital problems." Furious arguments erupted over one issue: my husband insisted that we begin using contraceptives again.

"How can we think of having a child," he said again and again, "if we have such serious problems with our marriage?"

If we used contraceptives, there was no chance for a pregnancy, and consequently there could be no infertility problem. Or, even surer, if we did not have intercourse, we certainly did not have an infertility problem. And, surest of all, if we got a divorce, we clearly had no infertility problem. It became almost easier for us to contemplate divorce than to face the fact of infertility.

You may not reach this extreme, but you will undoubtedly want to rationalize your situation at the outset. If millions of couples in the United States have no problem, why should you? You may have put off having children for a few years while you were getting settled in your marriage or your careers. You had heard all about getting pregnant by accident, so you compulsively chose a method of contraception. One day the time seems right to begin your family and you stop using any birth control method. Or you have gotten married with the idea you will begin your family right away. In either case, once the decision is made, you probably smile at each other, count ahead nine months, and imagine taking care of a sweet little baby just a year from now. But the first month you, the woman, menstruate. Another month goes by, and you menstruate again. You both begin to wonder what is wrong. People tell you not to worry. Someone tells you about Great Aunt Samantha who took two years to conceive her first child. Or about someone else who had a child after twelve years of marriage. Terrific. You groan, imagining yourselves twelve years older. The next month and the month afterward pass and still no pregnancy. When do you decide you have a problem?

Since the standard medical definition of infertility is the failure to conceive a child after one year of intercourse without contraception, many doctors advise waiting that year before initiating an infertility workup. In the past some doctors even advised waiting two years. Physicians have good reasons for suggesting that you wait a year. Some couples (about 17 percent) simply take six to twelve months to conceive.[1] In fact several experts mention many cases in which a patient's first or second appointment for an infertility evaluation is canceled because the couple has found out they are going to have a baby.[2] But, if you decide to wait a year, wait patiently.

If you find that tension and anxiety are overwhelming, you may want to initiate an evaluation sooner than a year. If you constantly try to estimate the day of ovulation and force intercourse then, you will turn an expression of love into a mechanical and even hostile act. You may find yourselves dreading intercourse. Or you may avoid it altogether, as we finally did. You may find that your life is filled with fears about what is wrong. Actively seeking help, merely knowing you are doing something about the problem, may be a relief.

Tension and anxiety are not the only reasons to begin thinking about starting an infertility investigation before a year goes by. There are several other reasons for beginning a workup after only six months of trying.

For a woman the first reason is age. This important fact is well known in medical circles, but not commonly known or understood by the general public. Female fertility decreases with age, particularly after the age of thirty-five. A classic study by Dr. Christopher Tietze, now of the World Population Council, has indicated that one in ten previously fertile women will be infertile by the age of thirty-five, one in three by age forty, and seven in eight by age forty-five.[3] Couples who have deliberately put off having children or couples who marry relatively late in life may want to begin an infertility workup before a year of trying to conceive goes by. Dr. Melvin Taymor of the Harvard Medical School insists that a woman over thirty-five should *definitely* begin a workup after only six months of trying to conceive.[4]

There is still another reason to initiate an infertility workup before a year goes by. If a woman has been using the pill as a means of contraception and then discovers she is unable to conceive on going off it, she should seek help early. For many years doctors have been aware of problems with ovulation following the use of oral contraceptives, the birth control pills.[5] But the advantages of effective contraception have been thought to outweigh the disadvantages suffered in only a small percentage of cases.

You all know that birth control pills are effective because they interfere with ovulation. But do you know that some researchers have found that in 20 percent of cases ovulation may not resume until three months after discontinuation of the pill? [6] In a smaller percentage of cases, 2 to 5 percent, they have found that it may take a year for ovulation to return.[7] The reasons for this are by no means clear to the medical profession. Some doctors feel that a woman will revert to whatever pattern of ovulation she had before using the pill: if she did not ovulate before, she may not ovulate afterward. The experts argue that the pill does not cause infertility in these women, but rather it masks problems with ovulation that existed previously. Some specialists feel that problems with ovulation following the pill may be an advantage for infertile women, because such problems force these women to discover and investigate them sooner.

It is important to stress that treatment is available to restore or induce ovulation, and that the sooner treatment is initiated the better. It is also important to stress that birth control pills have *not* been related to other causes of infertility. If a woman goes off the pill and then discovers problems with her fallopian tubes, with her cervix, or other problems unrelated to ovulation that render her infertile, she should not blame the pill.

Above all, it is important to decide as a couple when you want to undertake a thorough infertility investigation. You are the best judges of your particular situation. You can best assess the level of your anxiety. Infertility is a couple's problem, one of the few medical disorders that is shared by two people.

Both of you should be ready to undergo testing and examination, for no infertility workup is complete or valid without the participation of the two partners.

The mere decision to begin an investigation may be a relief, but it is not a guarantee that your troubles are over. You must be sure you are receiving a thorough evaluation. You must be sure you are in good hands.

CHAPTER 5

Where Do You Go for Help?

A JOINT BIRTHDAY celebration is an unlikely place for major
medical decisions, and we certainly had not planned on making
any. After the trials of the preceding years — a near miss
divorce and a somewhat shaky truce — we looked forward to
forgetting problems with friends from out of town whom we had
not seen in years. I had grown up in the mid-West with Anne.
Our Scorpio birthdays had been a secret bond in school days
and, when both of us had married Scorpios, the bond became
even tighter. We had talked for years about celebrating our
birthdays together, and finally a business trip had brought Anne
and Greg north in November.

Since we were all Scorpios, we knew we were bon vivants
and as self-centered and egotistic as Narcissus. It was easy to
laugh as we recognized ourselves in the horoscope that a com-
puter in Grand Central Station had spit out for me. Avaricious
. . . self-centered . . . difficult to live with. My eyes met my
husband's wryly understanding gaze. I continued to read down
the page, and then I stopped.

"Well, this one's accurate for *us*," I said grimly. " 'Health
problems: diseases of the genital and sexual organs.' "

"But that one is true for us, too," Anne, the mother of two,
asserted. "Didn't you know? It took us years to have our first
child."

And so the opening was made. For months we had talked about our problem with scarcely anyone but family and doctors. The birthday party became a recital of infertility woes. We talked about what tests had been performed, how equivocal the results seemed to us.

"We are at an impasse now, and we just do not know what to do," I said. "My gynecologist insists that the sperm count is the problem. But the urologist says it is within normal limits."

"They told us that, too," my friend wailed sympathetically.

"The gynecologist thinks all my test results are normal," I continued. "But I know that my reactions to one of the tests are not like what I've read in textbooks. And what's more, the gynecologist says he does not recommend any more tests for me."

Our friends jumped in. "But there *are* other tests. You must go to see a specialist. We started with a generalist gynecologist when we were living out west. He thought everything was fine with all the female factors, and that it was possibly a problem with the sperm count. But when we moved back to the mid-West, we went on to endocrinological experts, and they found the problem. They were the only ones who could give me that experimental fertility drug to make me ovulate. The generalist gyns are good, especially if your problems are relatively simple. But they just do not see a tremendous number of very complex cases of infertility."

My husband and I had talked about it before. Because it was hard for us to decide we had a problem, it was difficult to decide we needed a specialist. We were also hesitant about leaving a good doctor. We knew he had treated other cases of infertility. A friend of mine had seen him and had gotten pregnant after just seven months. But perhaps her case was less complicated than ours. Her husband's sperm count was "zillions," according to both of them. And she had gotten pregnant the same month her "tubes got blown," as she said. Maybe our case was more difficult. We decided that night to go to a specialist.

*

There are many kinds of doctors you might see when you discover you have a problem. Like us you may be already seeing a generalist ob-gyn or a family doctor. You may feel perplexed about the number of different kinds of doctors. Who are they? What is their experience with infertility? Which one should you see?

The Doctors Who Might Treat Infertility

The Family Doctor

Family doctors are usually general practitioners or internists who offer general medical care for all sorts of health problems. When they feel that your problem requires more specialized care, they usually refer you to a specialist.

Both the general practitioner and the internist learned something about infertility in medical school. But they probably have very little formal training in dealing with the problem. They can perform some of the basic tests, such as the sperm count, the thyroid tests, and the basic physical and sexual examinations. They can be helpful in providing information about conception and in referring you to a doctor who has been trained in infertility if your case seems difficult to resolve.

The Obstetrician-Gynecologist

Ob-gyns, as they are commonly known, are specialists in pregnancy and in women's diseases. They have had three to four years of residency training in obstetrics and gynecology. This training is not limited to instruction in the delivery of babies. The ob-gyn also learns preventive medicine-health maintenance of healthy women; contraceptive measures; prenatal care; how to treat problems in pregnancy; how to diagnose and treat various diseases of the female genital organs; and gynecological surgery. Training in treating infertility is included, but only as one part of the program. Generalist ob-gyns have learned the tests for infertility and the treatment of infertility problems, but they usually devote only part of their practice to these problems. Ob-gyns who make a special study of infertility become subspecialists in that field and will be discussed below.

The Urologist

Urologists are specialists in diseases of the genitourinary system — the kidneys, the bladder, and urinary tract — in both men and women, and specialists in the reproductive system in men. They have had five years of residency training, two in general surgery and three in urology. Their training includes: basic surgery and surgery for urologic problems; how to diagnose and treat diseases of the genitourinary system; and how to evaluate and treat infertility in men. As in the case of the ob-gyn, training in treating infertility is only one part of the total training program. The average urologist, like the average ob-gyn, devotes a comparatively small amount of his practice to treating infertile men.

Subspecialists in Infertility

Certain doctors devote extra time to studying infertility and become subspecialists in the field. These physicians are usually ob-gyns, but several noted subspecialists in various aspects of infertility are urologists, endocrinologists, and anatomists. Some of these doctors become ''sub-subspecialists''; that is, they become experts in one area of infertility, for example, the glandular problems that cause infertility in women. But whether they have special interests or not, they know a great deal about all phases of infertility and they see a great number of cases. Only a few doctors devote their entire practice to infertility, however.

The Infertility Clinic

Most university and teaching hospitals have infertility clinics, which are generally associated with the departments of obstetrics and gynecology and run by doctors with a particular interest and expertise in infertility, usually subspecialists in infertility. They are also the training ground for future subspecialists in infertility.

These clinics have the advantage of providing you with a host of doctors interested in infertility. Because they are located within a hospital, they provide you with easy access to specialists in other related fields, such as urology, endocrinology, and radiology. They also have the added advantage of almost always being open to all patients regardless of their economic situation. Some of these clinics have a sliding scale of fees that makes treatment available for almost everyone.

Since infertility specialists and clinics are limited in number, how can you locate them? There are a variety of ways. Your own doctor could refer you to a clinic or specialist. If you do not have a family doctor, you could contact the local office of Planned Parenthood, an organization which provides services for infertile as well as fertile couples. A few offices of Planned Parenthood have infertility clinics; others counsel you and refer you to a clinic or specialist in the area.

If you do not have access to an office of Planned Parenthood or to a doctor who can refer you, you can still locate a clinic or specialist on your own. Contact nearby university medical schools or teaching hospitals. The university medical center near us lists a separate number for its infertility department in the telephone book. If you are not near a medical school, you may write to the American Fertility Society (1608 Thirteenth Avenue South, Birmingham, Alabama 35205). This is an organization of over five thousand doctors interested in the problem of infertility. The organization publishes an annual directory, where you can find the names of member doctors in your area who deal with the problems of infertility. Local groups for people with infertility problems are beginning to appear in certain areas, and these groups might be able to help you locate a doctor. A few of these organizations are listed on page 170.

Which Doctor Do You Choose?

As you can see, there are many kinds of doctors who treat infertile patients. Which doctor should treat you? A family doctor could be consulted for the most basic tests, but if your case is complicated, you should ask him or her to refer you to a specialist. If you do not have a family doctor, you have two alternatives. Either you can go directly to an infertility specialist or clinic where you will be treated as a couple (there are many sound arguments for doing this) or you can go to a team, a generalist gynecologist for the woman and a urologist for the man.

The Infertility Specialist or Infertility Clinic

Several experts recommend that you begin with an infertility specialist or clinic.[1] My husband and I agree, after our experience with a series of doctors. There are several good reasons.

A specialist or clinic works every day with infertility problems. Yours can thus be put into better perspective, judged against the thousands of other cases already treated.

Your case will always be seen as a couple's problem. Coordinating the gynecologic evaluation of the woman and the urologic evaluation of the man is part of the daily experience of a specialist or clinic. A gynecological specialist is accustomed to working closely with a urologist on this problem. In a clinic the two will often be working under the same roof. In either case, the doctors can construct a picture of you as a couple.

A clinic or a specialist has daily experience in treating complicated problems. You will probably be able to receive both diagnosis and treatment from the same doctors, rather than finding out from one doctor that your problem is so complex it must be treated by a different doctor who is an expert. You begin where you might well end up.

Finally, specialists and clinics work on the assumption that everything is not normal if the couple does not conceive a child. They exhaust every possibility in looking for the cause. They must come to terms with all factors involved.

Our long experience with infertility taught us the importance of these arguments. We know well the importance of a specialist's daily experience with infertility problems. Two of the generalist gynecologists we saw evaluated the sperm count as the single contributing cause of our infertility. We were dismayed because we knew that in most cases a low sperm count is difficult to treat. We were also puzzled because the urologist maintained that the count was within normal limits. When we finally saw an infertility expert, he immediately found the sperm count low but judged it perfectly adequate in light of his experience with others.

We also know well the importance of close coordination of the investigations of male and female. Before we got into the hands of an infertility expert, my generalist gynecologist and my husband's urologist each insisted that the other should continue looking for the cause or cure.

In our case, much important time was lost looking for the right specialist. Had we begun there, we would have gotten to the root of the problem sooner. Instead, once the generalists had focused on a low sperm count, finding no obvious problem with me, they assumed that the rest of the female factors were normal and did not complete my evaluation. This was a mistake, on our part as much as on theirs. We should have insisted, because a high percentage of cases have multiple factors involved. Moreover, time is of the essence. An undiagnosed disease, such as my endometriosis, can only get worse.

The Team: Gynecologist and Urologist

The number of infertility specialists and clinics is limited. So your study may well begin with a gynecologist and a urologist. If your problems are relatively simple, you may find the solution there. But if you do begin with a gynecologist and a urologist, you should be aware of certain important demands to make.

Make certain that your doctors are truly working together. They may not necessarily be in partnership, or even have offices in the same building, but they should work in close consultation with each other. If at the end of the preliminary workup the male factor seems questionable, ask for a joint interview with both urologist and gynecologist to assess the situation. If there is disagreement between the two doctors, you should get a second or third opinion.

Be sure that your doctors have a specific timetable in mind. Infertility experts suggest that a thorough basic examination should take from four to eleven months to complete.[2] It takes this long because several of the tests must be performed at specific times in the woman's menstrual cycle. Because we did not have a definite timetable, our initial investigation dragged on for eighteen months.

Make certain that you and your doctors assess the situation thoroughly at the end of the basic investigation. You should be sure you both understand what tests have been performed and why; what the results show and where your results deviate from the norm; what tests and treatments should be prescribed now. Ask about further procedures. There are some that make possible a more complete examination of the female pelvic organs, either with x ray in hysterosalpingography or directly with a telescopelike device in culdoscopy or laparoscopy. (See pages 81–84.) If the doctors cannot pinpoint a specific cause, these tests must be performed in order that the investigation be complete. Immunologic testing is also important, so ask about its availability in your area. Do not let the medical terminology scare you. Be secure in your knowledge. It was I who suggested and then insisted that hysterosalpingography be performed.

If your case seems difficult to resolve, you may find yourself eventually in the hands of an infertility specialist. You may end up where you could have begun. Your doctor may refer you to a specialist. Or you may decide to refer yourself to another doctor. When should you make this decision? How should you proceed?

Consulting a Second or Third Doctor

If you encounter conflicting opinions, you should consult another doctor. If you feel that all questions have not been answered, you should consult another doctor. If you know that there are tests which have not been performed, you should consult another doctor. If we had not had the sense to question, we would not have a child today.

If you do consult a second or third doctor, you should expect another thorough examination. You should expect a complete history and a complete physical examination. You should expect the doctors to repeat certain tests. They will do this to check for themselves the results which others have reported. If the tests are not repeated, you should be sure that the earlier test results and X rays are thoroughly reevaluated. You should expect — and demand — all of these procedures. It is entirely possible that something may have been missed or misinterpreted in the first investigation. Make sure your second or third doctor proceeds completely and thoroughly.

The last doctor I saw was the only one to ask to see the X rays which the first doctor had taken at my insistence.

"But the doctor said the X rays were normal," I said. "And the other doctors I saw did not want to see them — even the one specialist I consulted briefly." The doctor nodded his head, as if he had heard this response a thousand times. "Yes," he said, "I understand. But I still want to see the films for myself."

I obtained the X rays, not without some difficulty, and hand-delivered them to my doctor. After only a moment's perusal, his experienced eyes immediately picked up kinking and possible adhesions of the fallopian tubes, a diagnosis missed by the first doctor and never considered by the others I had consulted since they had not seen the X rays for themselves.

Whether you go to a specialist or a generalist, you yourself must become an expert. Know what the essential tests are and make sure you have all of them. Know what the standard results are, so that you can understand your own results. Know what further tests and treatments are available.

Send for the basic information put out by Planned Parenthood, The Barren Foundation, or the American Fertility Society.[3] Read the most recent books written about infertility, some of which are listed in the bibliography on pages 187–88. You may even want to look at certain key medical works. You must understand what is being done and why. You will be more relaxed if you do understand. And you will be able to judge what kind of an investigation you are receiving. It is essential to know what constitutes a thorough and complete infertility investigation. You deserve one, and so do the other five million infertile couples.

CHAPTER 6

What Are Your Responsibilities?

YOU HAVE DECIDED to undertake an infertility investigation. You have been able to locate a doctor. You may feel that now it is the doctor's responsibility to make a diagnosis and cure you. This is not entirely correct. You too have important responsibilities. What are they?

Your Medical History

You have lived with yourself longer than anyone else has. You know your body better than anyone else can. It behooves you to think carefully about your medical history, to remember all you can, and to tell the doctor everything in as straightforward a manner as possible. If you are unsure about which childhood diseases you had, find out. If you think you will not be able to remember all the details — names of drugs, dates of childhood diseases, onset of symptoms — make a list and take it with you. Do not feel self-conscious about it. It will help you, and in turn your doctor.

A Complete Evaluation

Commit yourself to a thorough evaluation. Make certain that both you and your spouse are tested completely. Persist until you feel all questions have been answered.

Be honest with your doctor. If you have been pregnant before, if you have had an abortion, say so. One friend of mine was embarrassed about this and concealed it from her doctor, withholding a very important clue to the cause of her infertility.

Be honest on the tests. I know of one case in which a man hoodwinked his urologist on his sperm counts. Instead of bringing his own sperm for analysis, he brought in the sperm of a friend of his. He knew his own count was low, so he tried to save face this way. But what good did it do?

Above all, persevere. Try not to get discouraged as you go through the battery of tests. Insist that all tests be performed. If you are determined you want to continue, let your doctor know. One woman demanded that her doctors perform a certain treatment not once, but seventeen times! The doctors were skeptical that this persistence would pay off, but they acceded to her wishes. And they were overjoyed when the woman finally became pregnant.[1] There are a number of cases in the medical literature like that.

Expense

Inform yourself at the outset about the cost of tests and treatment. Fees vary from community to community. You might be able to obtain some idea of local standards from city or county medical societies, or there may be a directory for your community put out by consumer groups. You can certainly find out from your own doctor what his fees are. You can investigate the range of fees charged at infertility clinics. You may not need all the tests described in this book. You may find a solution early. But it is wise, at the outset, to have a realistic notion of what the complete workup could cost.

If you go to a subspecialist, you should expect higher fees, but there is good reason for this. You are paying for more than just a test or a treatment. You are paying for the doctor's experience. A specialist who has performed a procedure several hundred times has had more experience than others who perform it only infrequently. Moreover, having seen many hundreds of cases of infertility, the specialist is better able to judge just where you fit into the total picture of infertility. A generalist ob-gyn may be able to perform certain tests perfectly adequately — but how will the results be interpreted? In our case, the infertility subspecialists gave entirely different interpretations to tests that had been interpreted negatively by the generalists. An expert's eyes, hands, and past experience seemed worth the money to us. Remember, too, that subspecialists are associated with the infertility clinics of teaching hospitals, where treatment is usually available to everyone regardless of economic situation.

PART THREE

What Constitutes a Thorough Evaluation?

What is the matter with us? Why can't we have a baby? Whose fault is it? Who is to blame?''

Questions like these flood over you at the beginning of your investigation. You are naturally anxious. You are uncertain about what will be found; you are afraid it is your fault. You wonder how your spouse will feel if it is your fault. Above all, you do not want to be told that you will never be able to have a child.

These are normal worries. But you should make a superhuman effort to dismiss the notion of fault or blame. Fertility is a condition shared by a couple. After all, a woman cannot get pregnant by herself. Moreover, fertility is a relative matter. Superfertility in a male may make up for subfertility in a female — and vice versa. There is one important reason for correcting every problem. But there are other reasons as well. Because more than one factor is at work in a large number of couples with infertility, you should make sure that your workup is as thorough as possible. All tests should be performed to rule out every possible malfunction in both male and female. All conditions should be treated. Because infertility is a couple's problem, the basic minimum workup must include an examination of each partner.

CHAPTER 7

Basic Preliminary Workup of the Woman

THE BASIC workup for the female is more lengthy than the male's because there are more functions that should be tested. All of the tests in the basic workup can be performed in the gynecologist's office (or in a laboratory in the case of blood and urine studies). One of the tests is even charted by the woman at home. Several of them must be timed to coincide with certain days in her monthly cycle, so the testing cannot be concluded in one or two visits. However, all of these preliminaries can be performed over a four- to six-month period, and experts recommend that the basic investigation should not be stretched out longer than that.

I had some of the basic tests without really knowing it. On that first regularly scheduled visit, my gynecologist asked the routine questions in a standard health and sexual history. He performed a pelvic exam, taking the usual Pap smear. And he assured me that three months of trying to conceive was not really enough of a trial.

"Perhaps you're just missing the right day," he said, reinforcing our rationalizations.

"Should I start making a temperature chart?" I asked. I had read about the charts years earlier when my husband had done a clerkship in ob-gyn, so I knew how the charts could indicate the presence or absence of ovulation.

"You could, if you really want to," the doctor answered. "But personally, I think it's a bit early for that. If nothing happens in a few months, come back and we'll see what we can do to help."

So the official investigation began for me a few months later when I returned, armed with the temperature charts which I had made on my own initiative.

After looking these over, the doctor said the charts looked good. He leaned across the desk to show them to me, saying, "See, in the first part of your cycle your temperature runs low. Then, around day sixteen, there's a marked shift upward. That indicates that your cycle is definitely biphasic, and it's a pretty good sign of ovulation."

I looked politely at the charts, but I had already figured out that the temperature record was biphasic. I had been poring over the charts for weeks.

"However, just to be sure of ovulation, I'd like to do an endometrial biopsy," he continued. "That has to be performed on the first day of the menstrual cycle. So you'll have to come back when you get your period next. You just got your period today? What a coincidence! Come on into the examining room."

Without even planning, I had hit the right day. The infertility investigation had begun!

Your investigation will probably begin with the infertility problem firmly established in your mind. And you will probably start at the beginning, with a detailed history and physical exam.

Essential Tests in a Basic Investigation

Detailed History and Physical Examination

The doctor should take a complete medical history, asking you questions about many aspects of your health, both past and present. A complete physical examination should also be performed, including a chest x ray. Did you ever have suspected appendicitis or bouts of unexplained abdominal pain? When did these occur? Did you ever have abdominal surgery? When? What kind was it? Were there any complications? Is there a family history of tuberculosis? Is there a family history of infertility? Any aunts or uncles, great-aunts or great-uncles who also had problems having children? It is well known that a ruptured appendix, genital tuberculosis, or infection after pelvic surgery can damage the fallopian tubes. The physician should even ask you about poor tolerance of cold weather, as this may indicate a malfunctioning of the thyroid gland, which can play a role in infertility.

Menstrual and Sexual History

This is a very important part of the workup, so make every effort to be accurate and precise. How old were you when you began to menstruate? What is the length of your menstrual cycle? (Do not be confused about how to count the days. Remember, day one is the first day bleeding begins, and the last day — day twenty-eight or thirty or whatever — is the day before bleeding begins again.) How many days does the bleeding last? How regular are your cycles? Are they always the same number of days long or do they vary from month to month? Have you ever had prolonged cycles, of up to forty or fifty days, for example? Have you ever gone through several months without menstruating? If so, when? Do you have pain with menstruation? Have you noticed any change whatsoever in your menstrual flow? More blood? Less blood? Has there been more pain, or pain of a different character? If you normally have a high tolerance of pain, let your doctor know so that your pain can be more accurately interpreted. I knew I was experiencing more severe menstrual cramping than I had previously; this is a common symptom of endometriosis. But since I have a high tolerance of pain and could control the discomfort with aspirin, the doctor discounted the significance that I attached to the pain. I should have insisted more firmly.

Be frank in discussing your sexual history. Gonorrhea and aseptic abortions are two of the prime causes of damage to the fallopian tubes; any history of these should be mentioned. Be prepared to answer questions about your sex life. These are as essential to a thorough evaluation as a physical examination. What method of birth control have you used? If you are taking the birth control pill, know which kind and what dosage; do not simply talk about the red ones or the blues ones. How frequently do you have intercourse? Have you been compulsive about douching immediately after intercourse? Have you noticed any changes whatsoever in the way you experience intercourse? Any discomfort? Any pain? How can you best describe it? Pain at intercourse, dyspareunia, is significant, especially if it leads you to avoid sexual encounter. Moreover, it usually indicates a significant physiological problem — in 85 percent of the cases, according to two experts, the late Sophia Kleegman and Sherwin A. Kaufman of the New York University Medical School.[1] You will probably be asked about orgasm. However, it is important for you to know that female orgasm is *not* necessary for conception.

Infertile couples always wonder about the relationship of their patterns of intercourse to their problem. Be honest about this. If you have intercourse only once or twice a month, you may be missing entirely any exposure during the fertile period. On the other hand, too frequent intercourse in an excessively zealous attempt to get pregnant can drastically lower an already low sperm count and thus affect fertility. "Saving up" sperm by abstaining from intercourse prior to your estimation of the fertile period may result in more sperm but can adversely affect their motility, the characteristic that many experts feel is the most important one for fertility.

Arising immediately after intercourse and douching after intercourse are clearly not effective contraceptives, but they may be significant in couples with borderline fertility. If these are your habits, you should tell your doctor. Physicians usually recommend the male superior position for ejaculation. They also advise that the woman remain flat on her back for at least thirty minutes after intercourse during her fertile period and they advise against the use of lubricants or douches.

All of this information is important for the infertility workup. The questions do not indicate prying on the part of the doctor. In fact, if doctors avoid asking you these questions, you should begin to wonder how comfortable they are with the problem. If there are difficulties communicating at the beginning of the investigation, think of the problems you may encounter later when you need clear answers and straight advice. Some women might intuitively choose this moment to consult another doctor.

Pelvic Examination

Most women are undoubtedly familiar with the pelvic exam in which the doctor examines the genital organs and looks at the vagina and cervix through a special instrument, the speculum. Many women find this examination uncomfortable, both physically and psychologically. Heightened reactions caused by anxiety may only increase your discomfort and mask pain caused by other factors. Help your doctor and yourself by learning techniques of relaxation for the pelvic exam as well as for the other tests you will be undergoing.

The physical examination of the female reproductive organs may reveal rare abnormalities of the vagina, cervix, or uterus, as well as infections of the vagina or cervix, benign tumors of the uterus, enlarged ovaries, or pain that could indicate problems in the pelvic cavity. Some of these problems can be treated immediately; others are like clues in a mystery that must be investigated further.

You should know that the fallopian tubes are so small that they cannot be felt on pelvic exam. Their shape and condition can only be thoroughly revealed by tests which allow the doctor to visualize them, either by x ray or directly by culdoscopy or laparoscopy. (See pages 81–84.)

Laboratory Studies of Blood, Urine,
and Thyroid Function Tests

These studies are performed in a laboratory on specimens taken there. They may uncover a variety of conditions such as hypothyroidism, an underfunctioning of the thyroid gland, which can play a role in infertility.

Tests to Determine Ovulation

If you do not menstruate, you are probably not ovulating. However, even if you are menstruating, you may not be producing eggs and ovulating. Hence, two tests are commonly used to determine whether ovulation is occurring or not, and a third test may be advised by your physician.

Basal Body Temperature Charts (BBT). These are daily records of the patient's temperature entered on a special graph (Fig. 5, following page 170). The chart covers the whole menstrual cycle from day one to the beginning of the next cycle. Then a new chart begins with the first day of menstruation as day one. The temperature is taken either orally or rectally for five minutes each morning, immediately on awakening and before any activity has taken place, and recorded on the chart. The patient also indicates any factors such as a cold that might affect the temperature. She also indicates when intercourse occurs. Charts of three or four cycles can reveal much important information.

In the first place, they can give some evidence about whether ovulation is occurring or not. Ovulation is indicated by a shift in body temperature around the middle of the month. In a normally ovulating female, the temperature will generally run several tenths of a degree higher in the second part of the cycle than in the first part of the cycle. This happens because the estrogen produced in the first part of the cycle lowers body temperature, whereas the progesterone produced in the second part raises it. In the first part, the temperature may run 97.4 F degrees or lower; in the second, 98 degrees or higher. Figure 5 shows a standard chart for a normally ovulating woman, but there are many variations in what is considered normal. For this reason it is essential that an expert interpret the charts to see if there is evidence of ovulation.

The charts can also indicate the presence of certain hormonal difficulties. A shortened second half of the cycle, the luteal phase, may reveal problems in the production of progesterone by the corpus luteum. This can prevent the growth of an adequate lining of the uterus. If an egg is fertilized, it will not succeed in implanting and will leave the uterus as an extremely early miscarriage, which may be interpreted as merely the next menstrual period. If the higher temperature lasts ten days or less, this kind of problem may be suspected.

Temperature charts should not be used to program intercourse. A sharp rise in temperature at midcycle is good presumptive evidence that ovulation has taken place. But it may be proof after the fact. The moment of ovulation as indicated by temperature changes has puzzled even the experts. The late C. Lee Buxton, Professor of Obstetrics and Gynecology at Yale University, and Earl T. Engle showed that ovulation could occur as many as forty-eight hours *before* the rise and as many as forty-eight hours *after* the rise.[2]

My specialist advised intercourse every other day starting on day eleven of a cycle one month, starting on day twelve the next month. Admittedly this *is* programmed performance, and some experts have reservations even about this.[3] And it does take some of the joy out of sex. I can remember thinking, "Oh, no, not tonight again!" But the regular alternation of days does keep you from constantly watching the slight rises and falls in temperature on your chart and trying to hit *the* one.

Endometrial Biopsy. This is another test to determine whether there is evidence that ovulation is taking place. It is performed in the gynecologist's office. Samples of the endometrium are scraped from several different places within the uterus with an instrument introduced into the uterus through the cervix. The samples are then treated and examined under a microscope to see if there is evidence that ovulation has occurred, and if enough progesterone has been produced to make a uterine lining adequate for the implantation of a fertilized egg.

The test is usually performed on the first day of the menstrual period, though some doctors recommend doing it three to four days prior to the onset of bleeding. A few experts feel that if the test is to be performed a few days before menstruation, you should use birth control measures during that month in order to avoid inadvertently interrupting a pregnancy which just happened to occur that month.[4] Others argue that the likelihood of interrupting a pregnancy is remote.

For this test you will assume the position used for a pelvic exam. The doctor secures the cervix, causing a slight pinching feeling, and then he scrapes off a bit of the uterine lining. I found I had cramping after the test, but other women experience little or no discomfort. Laboratory proof of ovulation and adequate progesterone production are worth whatever discomfort one has.

Vaginal Smears. Some physicians advocate a third test to help determine the presence or absence of ovulation.[5] During one cycle, samples of vaginal mucus are taken daily by the patient herself, fixed on glass slides, and kept in jars of a special solution. These smears can then provide a very accurate picture of daily hormonal changes during a given cycle, and some physicians feel that they provide the most precise indication of the time of ovulation. The study and interpretation of the smears is difficult and must be done by an expert. For this reason, vaginal smears are not always a standard part of the basic infertility workup.

CHAPTER 8

Two More Tests in the Basic Workup of the Woman

No ONE can fully describe what the tests will be like for you, but you may get some idea from a fuller account of my experiences with two of them — the Rubin test to determine tubal patency and the Sims-Huhner test to check on the viability of sperm, among other factors. You will see as well how widely the interpretations may vary.

"Hop on the table, Mary," the doctor said, jovially calling me by my first name as if we had been friends for years and had not just met that instant. My regular doctor had been called out of town unexpectedly, and he had referred me to an older colleague rather than put off the Rubin test yet another month. I was fascinated that the doctor looked almost exactly like Clark Gable, but his manner made me nervous.

"We'll just do this little test, and you'll probably get pregnant this very month. Then you'll know it was just all in your head. You'll wonder why you worried so much."

I stared at him in amazement, trying to understand why he was putting on this act. He busied himself with his instruments, whistling the way my father did when he was nervous. I wanted to counteract his overly casual manner. I told him that I had been very apprehensive about the test. I knew what a negative result would mean — total closure of the tubes — and I thought nothing could be done for that problem.

I was wrong on both counts, but the doctor did nothing to correct my misapprehensions.

Instead, he continued his patter. But he refused to meet my inquiring eyes, and a glimmer of sweat caught the light on his forehead. He knew what a negative result meant too, I thought.

I lay there, spread out in the standard gynecological pose, and I felt only a slight pinch as he secured the cervix firmly with an instrument in order to insert a small cannula or tube into the opening. I wondered when he would start to pass the carbon dioxide through the cannula. I had stopped listening to his continuous stream of talk and concentrated on what was happening, trying to hear the bubbles of gas above the pounding of my heart. Would the carbon dioxide go through my fallopian tubes? Would I feel any bubbling? What would the shoulder pain be like, the pain a friend had told me was so terrible? I focused my concentration, and I felt nothing.

"Well," he said, his voice cracking, "there's no evidence of passage of gas. Let me try once more."

I froze, and already my mind raced ahead to a hopeless conclusion. I felt so alone. What would I tell my husband out in the waiting room? Why did it have to be this? I was certain nothing could be done.

Failure on the second try. The doctor remarked that I seemed nervous, maybe that was the reason, and he left the room, mumbling, no longer so jovially, that he would talk to me in his office.

There, surrounded by his books, his diplomas and other certificates, his manner changed from overly casual to nervously serious. But it was I who initiated the conversation.

"What does it mean? Is there anything that can be done?"

He did not tell me that a negative result was often found on the first test, and that such a result was routinely followed by a repeat test.

Instead, he told me from deep in his throat, "Well, the only way to be sure is culdoscopy" — pause — "but the man who was a wizard at culdoscopy here . . . you saw him several years ago. Well, you know, he moved away a few months ago, and . . ." His voice trailed off as if culdoscopy had left town with the wizard. His moustache twitched slightly.

"If it is total closure of the tubes, and it, er, it looks that way . . . Well, some people might operate, but — well, the operations aren't usually successful . . . and there is always a risk in surgery. Well, I wouldn't want to say it's hopeless, but . . . Perhaps you should talk it over with your doctor when he returns from his trip."

Somehow I got out of his office. When I saw my husband in the waiting room, I couldn't talk.

"What is it?" he asked and continued to ask. I could only shake my head. My throat was tight and I felt I was going to suffocate. I almost hoped I would. It looked as if everything was over.

The next time I had the test was after I had had surgery. My specialist went about his business, with no mundane patter. Same pose, same pinch when he secured the cervix, same passage of gas. But a muted "Fine!" at the foot of the table.

"Really?" I said in disbelief.

"Sure," he responded, and as if to prove it, he shot another whoosh of gas through.

I sat up. The nurse asked me if I was all right. I started to say yes, and then it hit me. Storm troopers marching over my back. Slight dizziness. I lay down again, trying to rub the pain out of my shoulders. A wave of nausea passed over me, but I began to smile as I realized that the surgery had been a success: my tubes now really were open.

Rubin Test or Tubal Insufflation to Determine Tubal Patency

The Rubin test or insufflation of the tubes with carbon dioxide is a test to determine whether the fallopian tubes are open. It is performed in the gynecologist's office, usually on days six to twelve of the cycle. The timing is important, for it must be after the cessation of the menstrual flow and before ovulation. The doctor places a cannula in the cervix and then passes carbon dioxide through it into the uterus. If the fallopian tubes are open, the gas will pass out of the uterus through the tubes, and the doctor will note a drop in pressure on the pressure gauge. If the tubes are closed, there will be no passage of gas and no drop in pressure.

The procedure itself is not painful. But if the tubes are open and gas passes through, you should experience pain in one or both shoulders on sitting up after the test. The pain may be severe, as mine was when I got a double dose of gas, but it can also be milder. The important feature is that pain should occur immediately after the test, when you sit up. This is caused by the gas rising and being deflected by the diaphragm.

The first time I had the test, I felt no pain immediately afterward. But, a few hours later, I did experience mild shoulder pain. I reported this to the doctor, who interpreted it as evidence of passage of gas. I later found out that delayed shoulder pain sometimes occurs, but it does not always indicate that the tubes are clearly open. Instead it may indicate, as it did in my case, that the tubes are kinked up and hence not freely patent.

A clearly positive result on the test can provide valuable information — the tubes are open. Or at least one of them is. You can go on to the next tests.

A negative result, however, can have any number of meanings. You may have had temporary spasm of the fallopian tubes. Buxton and Southam found that over 35 percent of women with negative results had no evidence whatsoever of tubal problems when a more accurate test, the hysterosalpingogram, was used.[1] These women apparently had temporary tubal spasm during the test, a not uncommon occurrence.

A negative test can also indicate that adhesions or kinking interfere with the patency of the tubes. The tubes may be open, but they are so kinked up that gas cannot readily pass through. Nor can sperm or egg.

Finally, a negative test can indicate total closure of the tubes, but this does not help the doctors locate just where the blockages are located.

Because of the variability of the results, some physicians prefer to skip the Rubin test and proceed directly to a more reliable test, hysterosalpingography, described on pages 81–82.[2] Other doctors feel that one should begin with the Rubin test because it is relatively simple, it can be performed in the gynecologist's office, and it sometimes seems to clear the tubes so that the patient can become pregnant following the test. It worked this way for a friend of mine.

Whatever the specialists may argue, you should know that a negative Rubin test does not present a clear picture of hopelessness. You may be one of the women with temporary spasm of the tubes. But if a repeated test shows another negative result, you should insist on the more accurate hysterosalpingography, as I did. It can provide a much clearer picture of the problem. And if the results of the further tests reveal problems with the tubes, you should know that treatments are available for many of the problems and that they promise varying degrees of success.

Even if your Rubin test is positive and all other preliminary tests are normal, you may still not become pregnant. What do you do then? Do not stop looking. You should definitely go on to the other tests anyway — hysterosalpingography, culdoscopy, or laparoscopy. It is true that a positive test result does indicate tubal patency, but the patency may be in only one tube. Or kinking or adhesions of the tubes may prevent the egg and sperm from meeting. Or else the openings of the tubes may be so abnormally small that the normal process of picking up the egg is impeded. All of these conditions cannot be determined by the Rubin test. They can show up in other tests described on pages 81, 83–84.

2.

The day was honeysuckle hot with billows of clouds in an August sky as we drove north to the retirement home of an eminent infertility specialist. After two frustrating years of conflicting opinions, we had researched the medical literature, found an experienced specialist, and written a desperate, end-of-the-line letter. The famous physician had generously agreed to see us. So that day we were making a journey of several hours to be evaluated by an expert, to have a postcoital test performed by a master. He had advised us to time the test around the temperature rise charted by me. We had made love at six in the morning, and I had stayed on my back for one hour before we left.

I dreaded having the test performed again, not because of any pain involved (there is none), but because I did not want to hear the same negative results pronounced that I had heard before.

I remembered that first test well, even though eighteen months had passed since it was performed. The doctor had taken a sample of cervical mucus and had murmured some of his findings as he peered over his microscope. Then he had talked to me in his office.

"Well, it's not good," he said. "Five to ten sperm per high-powered field. We usually like to see twenty. And in some fields I found none. Let's see — your husband's sperm count?" He consulted the records, frowned, and continued.

"Well, you know, in school we learned the rule of sixes — sixty million per milliliter, sixty percent motility, sixty percent normal shape or morphology. In your husband's case, he only has twenty million per milliliter. It just seems too low."

Exasperated, I held my tongue. Both the doctor and I already knew the sperm count was in the low range of normal. Clearly we could not expect the test results to appear perfect. What I wanted to know was what the test results meant in our particular case. The doctor talked on and on. For him the test result was not a standard one: my husband's count did not conform to the mystical rule of sixes, therefore it was not normal.

"Well, you know there's very little that can be done about a low sperm count — *You* seem to be just fine, though."

Now the pines of the Adirondacks flying past the car windows brought me back to the present. We were almost there. As we drove up to the house, we saw a giant of a man with a shock of gray hair in the doorway. Greeting us warmly, he invited us in, wondering how we had found our way to him. We glanced at each other in amazement: he was one of the most eminent researchers in reproductive biology, having published and made important discoveries in this field for over forty years.

After a careful review of my charts and a careful history from both of us, he focused on my husband's habit of taking prolonged hot baths to relieve a low back problem.

"You really should avoid those hot baths," he said. "You know, excess heat can drastically lower a sperm count." And standing up, he demonstrated exercises for the back which could be done in a hot shower. Here was a physician treating the whole problem rather than just isolated factors.

The postcoital test was performed in his bedroom. I lay across his bed and looked around at the family pictures on the walls, the books on the bedside table. My husband held my knees, and the doctor put on a hat with a light that looked like a miner's helmet. He peered inside. "Ah, yes, fine." He put a drop of cervical mucus on a glass slide and handed it to my husband, then proceeded to do a pelvic exam. The lawn mower buzzed in the background.

He had put us both at ease, but I held my breath as he strode to his desk to bend over the microscope he had used as a medical student some fifty years ago. After what seemed a long pause, he said, "Per — fect!" — drawing out the syllables to emphasize his pleasure. I could not believe it.

"It's a grand specimen. Not quite so many as a sixty million man might have. But it is fine for you, just fine. Here, take a look."

My husband bent over the microscope, and I approached the desk.

"Can I look, too?" I asked. And there they were, tiny sperm cells swimming away. I moved the slide slightly. Still lots of sperm. I gasped.

We returned to the porch, and the doctor smiled at me. "Go ahead! Miss your period this month! Everything looks fine. Please miss your period!" And to my husband, "As far as I can see, everything seems healthy. But no one has actually looked inside. It could be a plumbing problem. Many of these so-called unexplained cases are, you know. At least, that's what I've found. I would say that culdoscopy is the next step. I'll refer you to my younger colleague who is an expert at that."

With this settled, we talked on his porch for a while about the pond he had constructed, about the chipmunks he had banded in order to trace their movements. As we prepared to leave, he took us around the side of the house to see his flowers.

"Look at this," he said. "Do you see this flower? It grows best in the shade. See, it produces this kind of leaf. But look here." He led us around to the front of the house. "In the sunlight, it has an entirely different response." He was as enthusiastic about the growth habits of these plants as he was about my getting pregnant, about anyone's getting pregnant. Even when my period came that month, we felt we were finally on the right road.

The Postcoital or Sims-Huhner Test

The postcoital test is performed in the gynecologist's office, timed to coincide with the fertile period of the cycle, around the time of the temperature rise. Your doctor will ask you to have intercourse during the preceding twelve hours, to remain in bed for at least half an hour afterward, and to avoid using any lubricants or douches. You should be sure to report how much time has elapsed since intercourse, since this may affect the interpretation of the test.

The procedure is absolutely painless. The doctor simply takes a large drop of mucus from the cervix, places it on a slide, and examines it under a microscope. He can then see how many sperm are there, and how well they are moving. Although this procedure can reveal much important information about the sperm, it should not take the place of a sperm analysis, which can reveal other problems and should be part of the standard evaluation of the male. (See pages 74–78.)

What can this procedure reveal? It can show the number of sperm that arrive at the cervix and their motility in the cervical mucus. It can also reveal certain qualities about the cervical mucus.

The test for the number of sperm is easy, but the results are not always absolutely black and white. There is a wide range of what is considered normal. Excellent results show twenty or more motile sperm per high-powered field of the microscope; six to twenty are generally considered good; one to five are fair.[3] If absolutely no sperm are present, the doctor should consider the problem of faulty coital technique as well as the problem of hostile cervical mucus in the female. The conditions of azoospermia and poor sperm motility may also be considered, if they have not already been discovered in a sperm analysis.

The test also reveals much about the characteristics of the cervical mucus.[4] At the time of ovulation, the mucus around the cervix changes from a rather heavy, viscous substance to a clear, shiny liquid resembling egg white. This type of mucus facilitates sperm survival and penetration. It is very alkaline and also extremely elastic. A test for this elasticity, or *spinnbarkeit* as it is known medically, can be performed at this time; the doctor simply measures the length the mucus will stretch before dropping onto a glass slide. The association of this elasticity with a woman's fertile period has been known about for centuries; it has been reported that primitive women test themselves for their most fertile period by stretching this mucus between their fingers. You too may have noticed an increased clear discharge around the time of midcycle, an indication of probable ovulation. Another test, the fern test, can be performed on the mucus at this time. If the mucus forms fernlike patterns when it is dried on a slide, it provides yet another indication of probable ovulation.

These three tests, the Sims-Huhner test, the test for elasticity, and the fern test, can tell much about the compatibility of sperm and mucus, about ovulation and the sperm count. They might also suggest that there are hormonal problems in the woman which affect the quality of the mucus, causing it to inhibit sperm movement (so-called hostile mucus).

As in the other tests, there is a variability in what constitutes normal in the postcoital test. If the results are fair, good, or excellent according to the standards mentioned above, there is always the possibility of pregnancy. It may take an expert's eye to put your particular test results in perspective, as it did in our case.

The eight tests described in this and the preceding chapter constitute the basic preliminary investigation of the female. To sum up, they are: detailed history and physical examination; menstrual and sexual history; pelvic examination; laboratory studies of blood, urine, and thyroid function; Basal Body Temperature Charts; endometrial biopsy; tubal insufflation (Rubin test); and postcoital test (Sims-Huhner test). A ninth test, the vaginal smear, is sometimes requested by some doctors.

The tests are designed to survey all aspects of a woman's reproductive capabilities. Is she in good health? Are her sexual organs mature and healthy? Is her sexual functioning normal? Is there a clear pathway from her vagina to the fallopian tubes for the sperm to travel? Does her vaginal and cervical mucus appear to be favorable to sperm? Is there evidence that she produces a viable egg? Are the tubes open to capture the egg, to allow the sperm to meet and fertilize the egg, and then to allow the fertilized egg to travel to the uterus? Is the lining of her uterus prepared to receive and nurture a fertilized egg? All eight of the tests should be performed, since several factors are often responsible for preventing conception. But the preliminary workup is not complete without an investigation of the male factors. Infertility is a couple's problem.

CHAPTER 9

Basic Preliminary Workup of the Man

THE MALE partner is an equal part of the couple. He should receive just as thorough an examination as the female, even though there are not quite so many tests to perform. The investigation of the male takes less time than the investigation of the female, but it is likely to be equally upsetting emotionally.

My husband looked grim the morning he was to have his first sperm count. "They'll probably find millions of dead sperm," he said glumly as he walked out the door. When he returned, he did not look much happier. I was afraid to ask what had happened.

"Well, it's within normal limits," he said. "Twenty million per milliliter. And five milliliters in all."

"That sounds good to me," I said. "Twenty million times five? A hundred million! That's an enormous number."

"Yeah, it's okay. But there's only fifty percent motility."

I did a fast calculation, dividing by two, and my heart sank. "What did the doctor say?" I asked.

"He said, 'lower limits of normal,' so I guess it's all right," my husband answered. But he looked downcast all the same. There was little I could do to cheer him up. This first sperm count had hit him hard. In spite of his medical training, he did not think ahead to other sperm counts nor did he think back to the other examinations he had gone through.

*

A single sperm count is not an adequate exam for the male because there are many factors that influence a male's fertility. Nor is the postcoital examination of the female, described on pages 69–70, a reasonable test of male fertility.

Essential Tests for a Man

Detailed history and physical examination

The doctor should perform a complete physical examination, including a chest x ray. It is extremely important that the penis and testicles be examined in a careful and detailed manner, with the patient standing and reclining. The prostate gland should be thoroughly palpated.

The doctor will also take a complete medical history. Have you ever had mumps? At what age? Was there an involvement of the testicles? Have you had gonorrhea or any other venereal diseases? Have you had any recent illness with a high fever? Is there a family history of tuberculosis? A family history of relatives with infertility problems? What is your consumption of alcohol, drugs, and tobacco? Are you taking any kinds of medication regularly? The doctor will also inquire about specific trauma of the genital organs; these include specific injuries, any exposure of the genitalia to x ray, and even prolonged exposure of the testicles to heat. As odd as it may seem, exposure of the testicles to heat can be produced by tight underwear, long hot baths, or even the confinement of driving too long in a truck or car.

This examination may uncover general health problems such as fatigue or poor diet, which can play a role in infertility. Past diseases can also adversely influence fertility: mumps orchitis in puberty or adulthood seriously damages the reproductive capacities of the testicles; gonorrhea and tuberculosis can damage the tubes in the testicles which carry the sperm out to the penis, as they damage the fallopian tubes in women; viral illness with a high fever can temporarily reduce the sperm count. Certain medications such as antimicrobial drugs, anticancer drugs, and some steroids can temporarily lower a sperm count. Individual sensitivities to alcohol, drugs, and tobacco can also affect fertility.

The examination of the genital organs may reveal that the testes have never descended into the scrotum or that they have not matured adequately. Varicocele, dilated testicular veins, may also be discovered; this condition affects the quantity and quality of sperm ejaculated. More rarely, malformations of the opening of the penis are discovered.

Sexual history

This should include questions about the onset of puberty as well as questions about sexual habits. The doctor should inquire about pregnancies in previous relationships. As in the female, this history may show an unconsummated marriage, impotence, or premature ejaculation outside the vagina, in addition to too frequent or infrequent intercourse. The doctor may also ask about masturbation. As mentioned before, ejaculation one or more times a day, whether by intercourse or masturbation, may actually lessen the number of sperm in each ejaculation. Since sperm can live between thirty-six to forty-eight hours, intercourse every other day is perfectly adequate.

Laboratory Studies of Blood, Urine, and Thyroid Function

As in the female, these tests, performed in a laboratory on specimens taken there, may uncover certain problems not revealed on physical exam, such as hypothyroidism, the underfunctioning of the thyroid gland.

Analysis of Sperm

This test is usually performed in the urologist's office. A sperm specimen is obtained by masturbation and placed in a clear glass container. This is the method of choice, but if a man is unable or unwilling to do this, he can obtain the specimen by using a special condom during intercourse.[1]

Specialists usually recommend that the test should be preceded by forty-eight hours of sexual abstinence, the length of time generally thought necessary to replenish an adequate supply of sperm. Others advise abstaining for as many days as are usual in a couple's normal sexual pattern, so that the specimen examined reflects the amount of sperm the woman is regularly exposed to. It is important to follow your doctor's suggestion in this matter.

The sperm are placed on a slide and examined under a microscope, where not only their number but also their quality will be revealed. The test results should include: the total number of milliliters per specimen; the number of sperm per milliliter; the percentage of sperm that are actually moving (motility); and the percentage that have a normal shape and size (morphology). Experts recommend that tests for these factors should be repeated several hours later on the same specimen in order to evaluate the life of the sperm.

It is also recommended that a second or third sperm analysis be made if the first one seems low. Many factors mentioned above can temporarily lower the sperm count. For example, viral illness with a fever a few weeks before the test can dramatically lower the count.

The analysis of the sperm can reveal much important information. If the single analysis or subsequent analyses do not fall within the limits of normal, the tests can show problems with number, motility, or morphology of the sperm as well as abnormalities of the liquid which carries the sperm.

The test can reveal oligospermia, an abnormally low number of sperm, or azoospermia, their total absence. If either of these conditions is found together with normal-sized testicles a testicular biopsy should be recommended. This test could determine if sperm are being produced inside the testicles but then prevented from leaving them by obstruction in the epididymis or vas deferens.

Problems with motility can be revealed in the analysis. These problems can range from a total lack of motility in all the sperm to motility in less than 40 percent of the sperm. The causes of low motility are poorly understood.

The analysis can reveal the presence of a high number of irregularly shaped sperm, or abnormal morphology. What causes their irregular shapes is still a puzzle to experts, and doctors cannot offer a cure for this. However, if the irregularity is immaturity and there are more than 4 percent immature sperm cells in the specimen, one expert suggests that the problem may be varicocele, which might not have been discovered on physical exam.[2]

Agglutination of sperm can show up in the test. Sperm may be present and active, but they clump together in groups and do not move freely. This may be caused by the fact that the male is allergic to his own sperm, a relatively rare condition the cause of which is still poorly understood. Or it may be caused by the deficiency of a certain agent which is normally present in semen to prevent agglutination.

The analysis can also show a reduced volume of semen. There are many active, normally shaped sperm, but the semen is reduced so that they have too little liquid to swim in.

Finally, the analysis can show a failure of the semen to liquefy. Normally, semen forms into a substance like jelly immediately after ejaculation and then liquefies in ten to twenty minutes. In some rare instances, the liquefaction does not occur and the sperm are thus trapped in a block of jelly, unable to move.

All these are abnormalities. Some of them can be treated with varying degrees of success.

But what is considered a normal sperm count? There is great variation in its definition. A few decades ago, researchers laid down the law that the minimum standards for male fertility were: 60 million sperm per milliliter; 60 percent normally shaped sperm (normal morphology); and 60 percent motility. This is the "rule of sixes" that one of my gynecologists was learning in a residency program in the mid-1960s. That this rule should still be taught today is amazing, since experts in urology have accepted quite different standards for male fertility for over two decades.

The experts in male infertility now think that the lowest limits of normal, the *minimum* standards are: 20 million sperm per milliliter; 60 percent normal morphology; and 40 percent motility.[3] These experts feel that the male can be ruled out as a significant factor in the couple's infertility if his count reveals 40 million sperm per milliliter; 70 percent normal morphology; and 40 percent motility. The sperm count that falls in the gray area between the minimum standards and those just cited may be considered as *one* of the factors in a couple's infertility, but their investigation should not stop there, as our initial one did.

John MacLeod, Professor of Anatomy at Cornell University Medical School and an expert in male infertility, has recently emphasized that motility seems to be more important than absolute number. Indeed, he vociferously urges continued investigation of the female if there are *any* active sperm present. His feelings are so strong that they are worth quoting:

> Indeed, the gynecologist again is urged to conclude his study of all aspects of the female side if the semen contains any *active* spermatozoa at all. If the experience of this reviewer is of any value, one certain truth in his 25 years of the study of human infertility is that normal pregnancies have and will occur in the chronic presence of appalling semen quality.[4]

To sum up, the essential tests for a man are: a complete medical history and physical exam; a complete sexual history; basic laboratory studies of blood, urine, and thyroid function; and one or more sperm analyses.

Occasionally the preliminary workups of both male and female uncover soluble problems which easily explain the infertility. An incorrectly consummated marriage or the inadvertent avoidance of intercourse at the time of ovulation can be remedied through education in sexual technique and physiology. An unconsummated marriage of long standing, premature ejaculation outside the vagina, or impotence can respond to psychotherapy of the behavioral model described by Joseph Wolpe or the direct behavioral couples technique developed by Masters and Johnson. Minor infections of the vagina and cervix can easily be treated. Any hypothyroidism in either man or woman can be treated with thyroid medication.

Sometimes a couple conceives during the course of the preliminary workup. The couple may simply have been one of those who require that long to conceive. Or, according to some doctors, insufflation of the tubes in the Rubin test may actually clear up minor problems in the fallopian tubes to facilitate conception.

If a fortuitous pregnancy has not occurred, you should meet with your doctors to assess the situation at the end of the preliminary investigation. If specific problems have been uncovered, treatment should be initiated. If questions of problems have been raised, further tests should be performed. If the tests show results that appear within the range of normal and pregnancy still does not occur, other tests should be performed.

CHAPTER 10

After the Basic Workup:
Evaluation and Other Tests

YOU BOTH have had the basic workup. There is still no pregnancy. It is time to meet with your doctors to assess the situation.

I remember the meeting we had with my gynecologist. A gray day, bitter cold. Christmas just a few weeks away. My doctor leafed through the charts, checking off the tests he interpreted as normal.

"Ovulation looks all right from the temperature charts. The biopsy showed a good rich uterine lining." Pause. "Thyroid all right."

We knew that. I asked him if it could be endometriosis.

"What?" he said. "What makes you ask that?"

"Well," I hesitated, "you know I've told you I think my cramps are different, more intense."

He looked back over a few pages. "No, I don't see any evidence of endometriosis."

"But something *has* to be wrong," I insisted. "What about the first insufflation your colleague did? I didn't feel the results were very positive," I said.

"Well, you remember, Mrs. Harrison, I performed that test again. And it seemed to me that at least *some* gas passed through."

I remembered the second test, but I felt the results had been just as negative as the first time. I did not argue that point. This conversation seemed to be becoming a battle of wills.

I said, "Well, I would be more convinced if I could have a hysterosalpingogram."

The doctor's blond eyebrows shot up in amazement. I did not even stumble over the syllables. My knowledge startled even me.

"Of course, if you insist. But it *is* expensive."

I started to muse on the price of knowledge — and health. The doctor was not finished, however. He rattled a few papers, as if to increase the drama, and then said, "Frankly, it is my opinion that it is a male factor."

What a Christmas present! The next consultation I made was with a psychiatrist.

My husband and I had arrived at the first impasse — a clear disagreement between my gynecologist and my husband's urologist. And we didn't have the sense even to ask for a consultation with both doctors. Every month, the rise in temperature occasioned frantic attempts on my part to get my husband into bed. And every month, menstruation brought with it a flood of tears, along with depression, guilt, anger. My husband attacked my sexuality; I attacked his masculinity. We both thought of divorce. And for a time, the evaluation ground to a halt.

In our case, the results of the preliminary workup clearly suggested further testing. A borderline sperm count, especially one that is defined as within normal limits by a urologist, should not be taken as the definitive answer. The questionable results of the tubal insufflation should have immediately led to other tests. I intuited this, and I began to insist on it.

So, in between consultations with a divorce lawyer and sessions with a psychiatrist to shore up my ego, I scheduled the hysterosalpingogram. I was sure something was wrong with me, and I wanted to find out what.

I had become a half-crazed fanatic. Why should I have the test when a divorce seemed imminent? My reasons still do not seem totally rational to me. If I could find out that something was wrong with me, I could take the burden of responsibility off my husband's shoulders. I might be able to find a cure. I might be able to produce a child for him. The divorce would be dropped. Or if nothing could stop the divorce, I might be able to find a cure anyway.

My husband fought the test, saying, "Why have it when we're not even trying to get you pregnant?" His ego was deflated, he had lost interest in the workup, and he was continuing to lose interest in me. However, he came to the hospital the day of the test. In retrospect, this was possibly the first turning point in our crisis.

The hysterosalpingogram was performed in the radiology department. It was painless, and in an hour I was on my way home. A gynecologist and radiologist worked together. I lay on an x-ray table and films were shot as a radio-opaque dye was infused through the uterus and tubes. When I heard the doctors remark that they saw spillage from the tubes on their special screen, I was relieved but puzzled. Maybe the tubes were open. At that point I did not understand that the X rays could be interpreted differently. It was not until several years later that the films were read as indicating possible adhesions.

Hysterosalpingography

This test is recommended for two reasons: if tubal problems are suspected after a negative Rubin test and if a patient has not become pregnant after a basic workup. It is performed after the cessation of menstrual bleeding and before ovulation occurs, between days six and twelve of the cycle.

The test can be very revealing. It can demonstrate that both of the tubes are open, when dye spills out from the tubes, and it can confirm that the uterus is normally shaped. Some authorities feel that it can occasionally be of therapeutic value. They report some pregnancies occurring in the month of the test or in the months following.

The test can also expose problems. It can show that one or both tubes are blocked and can pinpoint the area of obstruction. It can reveal kinking or adhesions of the tubes, as it did in my case. It can show anomalies of the uterus or tuberculosis, both rare conditions.

If the test reveals tubal problems or uterine anomalies, surgery can follow. In the unusual event that suspicion of tuberculosis is raised, further tests can be performed in that direction.

If the hysterosalpingogram seems normal an observation period can follow. But if pregnancy still does not occur, culdoscopy or laparoscopy *must* follow, and the sooner the better.

Other Tests of the Woman

Three other tests could be performed at this stage of the investigation, but there should be good evidence that they are needed.

Hormonal Studies

Special laboratory studies of steroids and gonadotropins in the female are indicated *only* in certain problems with ovulation. Certain of these tests are performed on a urine sample that consists of all urine excreted over a twenty-four-hour period. However, they are warranted in only 5 to 10 percent of cases of suspected ovulatory dysfunction.[1] In 90 to 95 percent of these cases, the Basal Body Temperature Charts and endometrial biopsy can provide adequate information on which to base hormone therapy.

Immunologic Testing

This procedure determines whether the woman is in some way allergic to her husband's sperm, a condition that is found only rarely. A blood sample from the woman is mixed with the man's sperm to determine compatibility. If the results suggest allergy, the physician can try to desensitize the wife to her allergy in a very simple manner. (See page 109.)

Culdoscopy, Laparoscopy, or Laparotomy

If there are normal findings in the earlier tests and pregnancy still does not occur, the final test of the female should involve visualization of the pelvic organs. This can be achieved by culdoscopy, laparoscopy, or laparotomy. In culdoscopy and laparoscopy, telescopelike instruments are inserted into the pelvic cavity to allow visualization. In laparotomy the abdomen is actually opened, so that direct visualization is possible. Recent improvements in the technical equipment for culdoscopy and laparoscopy make these the procedures used more often today.

Some physicians feel that these tests are the major diagnostic tool in an infertility workup, because only in these procedures are they actually able to look at the female's reproductive system. Moreover, unsuspected problems are discovered in 40 to 50 percent of the cases, according to Taymor.[2] Culdoscopy was the final test in my case, as I described in the prologue, and it was the only way my endometriosis was diagnosed.

Culdoscopy and laparoscopy are difficult procedures requiring an expert hand and eye, and the specialists themselves realize this. My husband's only exposure to culdoscopy had been as a medical student when he had assisted a professor of gynecology. "I could hardly see *anything* when the doctor let me look in the scope," he told me just before I was to undergo culdoscopy myself.

Both culdoscopy and laparoscopy are surgical procedures that require an overnight stay in the hospital. In both, a telescopelike device is inserted into the abdominal cavity so that the doctor can look directly at the ovaries, the fallopian tubes, and the uterus. In culdoscopy, the instrument is inserted through a slit cut in the vagina near the cervix. In laparoscopy, it is inserted through a small incision made in the abdomen. Local or spinal anesthesia is used for culdoscopy, whereas general anesthesia is usually used for laparoscopy. Since slightly different areas of the reproductive organs are visible in each of the procedures, physicians have argued about which is preferable.[3] Laparoscopy seems to be gaining popularity today.[4] However, in both procedures the doctor can see the ovaries, the fallopian tubes, and part of the uterus, and can test the patency of the tubes by passing dye through them to see if they are open.

These examinations can reveal: problems with the ovaries like multiple cysts or the formation of a hard outer shell; adhesions, which bind the ovaries or tubes to other organs; partial or total closure of the tubes; and diseases.

Endometriosis is one puzzling disease that may be discovered through culdoscopy or laparoscopy in women whose infertility has been unexplained up to that time. Since endometriosis and the other conditions mentioned above can exist with no symptoms at all, the direct visualization of the pelvis in culdoscopy, laparoscopy, or laparotomy is the only way to make the diagnoses.

Another Test of the Male: Testicular Biopsy

This test of the male should be used only in certain cases, when azoospermia or extreme oligospermia is associated with normal-sized testicles. It can be performed in the urologist's office under local anesthesia. The doctor takes a small slice of tissue from the testicle to determine if sperm are being produced there. The sliver is treated, placed on a slide, and examined under a microscope. If the slide reveals that sperm are being produced inside the testicle, blockage of the passages leading from the testicle to the penis may be suspected. Such a finding will indicate the need for an operation to open the closed passages of the testicle. Pregnancy has been reported following 20 percent of these operations.[5]

Testicular biopsy should not be performed routinely merely to make a diagnosis, but only if the urologist feels that it may reveal one of a few conditions that can be corrected surgically.

The Question of Psychogenic Infertility

In the course of your infertility workup, someone will probably tell you, "It's all in your head." Your parents, a well-meaning friend, a psychiatrist, a gynecologist. I heard it from a relative as well as from a psychiatrist. However, you should know that infertility experts are very cautious about making this diagnosis without fully testing both partners.

Buxton and Southam wrote in 1958 that ". . . the most significant areas in which psychological factors may affect fertility are impotence in the male and disruption of rhythmic pituitary-ovarian-endometrial relationships in the female." [6] In the preceding chapters you have read how psychological upsets can also cause premature ejaculation outside the vagina and ejaculatory incompetence in men, as well as frigidity in women. All of these conditions can be treated.

More recently, Melvin Taymor, Professor of Obstetrics and Gynecology at the Harvard Medical School, wrote ". . . more often than not the state of infertility and the diagnostic and therapeutic maneuvers involved are more likely to produce emotional factors than to have primary emotional factors produce infertility." [7] Other specialists agree, and they urge that all possible tests be performed in an effort to discover any possible physical cause.

Make certain that all of the tests that should be performed in a thorough infertility workup have been performed — and by an expert — before either of you is willing to accept a diagnosis of psychogenic infertility. If this diagnosis is made, ask for a clear explanation of exactly how psychological factors are causing your infertility. Is it impotence, premature ejaculation, or frigidity? Are there indications of a disruption of the hypothalamic-pituitary-ovarian relationship? If not, you may simply have a problem which lies beyond the realm of current knowledge about the causes of infertility.

CHAPTER II

The Emotional Burden of Infertility

THE BASIC infertility investigation described in Chapters 7–10 is a staggering array of tests and procedures, the result of years of research and experimentation. The tests are designed to investigate the myriad physical functions of the organs involved in the complex process of reproduction. After undergoing the tests, you both will feel that your bodies have been opened up and laid bare. Yet, while your bodies are subjected to the most elaborate of investigations to uncover the causes of your infertility, your minds may be left alone, to ponder and ruminate. There are no temperature charts to measure your emotional reactions to the investigation, nor is there any specific therapy for your anguish.

Even now, years later, I find the emotional side of infertility almost too painful to confront directly. In the preceding chapters, I have been able to share with you only isolated glimpses of my reactions — the anxiety and failure I felt when a psychiatrist suggested my infertility was psychosomatic, the hopelessness I felt when the first postcoital was negative, the emptiness I could not express when my gynecologist solemnly declared the problem was a male one and my husband's silent distance began, the panic and despair when my marriage threatened to dissolve. I have not even mentioned — and I hesitate to mention even now — the anger I felt at my husband when I allowed myself to believe the first gynecologist's interpretation of the data. Or later, the anger I felt at myself for believing him. I have not mentioned the stabbing envy I felt whenever I saw a pregnant woman, the tears that I could not stop when my sister brought her newborn son home from the hospital. Nor have I mentioned the horrifying metamorphosis of our love life into a chain of mechanical acts linked together only by the question: Will I get pregnant *this* time? Unhappiness was a constant during the investigation. Like the beating of a heart, it was always there, sometimes thumping, at other times barely audible, but always establishing the rhythm of my life.

The feelings which arose from infertility soon invaded the rest of my life, and they must have been more manifest than I can remember. I lost self-confidence; I felt I was no longer attractive. I was in a black mood, particularly when my period arrived after any slight delay, which I always interpreted as pregnancy. For me, the threat of divorce was a direct result of the infertility and a confirmation of my failure as a woman. For my husband, the more important factor seemed to be my steady loss of confidence and constant unhappiness.

How did we handle our problems? The best we could, but now it seems to have been more like just muddling through. The most significant mistake we made was not to proceed directly to the final tests with a specialist. Had we found the cause sooner, some of the anguish might have been avoided.

Anyone with infertility needs support, and in our protracted ordeal I was no exception. But where do you find it? I leaned heavily on my husband, so heavily that my dependence dragged him down. By nature reticent, I found it difficult to reach out to family or friends, to admit to outsiders that I had a problem, to seek their help. When I did reach out, it was like a child touching an animal for the first time, tentatively, with one finger, withdrawing at the very first negative reaction.

My family was loving, they let me know they cared, but could they really understand? During the first year of the investigation, they tended to fall prey to the same rationalizations that

I did. "You just must have missed the right time this month. You'll get pregnant next month." Neither of my sisters had infertility problems — one had timed the conception of her two children to the minute, the other seemed to become pregnant whenever her husband looked at her. In spite of their good will, they could scarcely fathom my problem, concerned as they were with avoiding another pregnancy. So I began to limit my solace-seeking to my mother, who had stopped worrying about birth control long ago and who seemed to be the only person during the whole ordeal who knew how much my heart ached.

When I turned, ever so tentatively, to friends, I found other difficulties. At best they offered nervous apologies or unsought medical advice. At worst they went beyond laconic apologies to outright blunders. My friend Gay meant well when she offered condolences about my problem. Always trying to look on the bright side, she went on without thinking, "Why, Mary, you don't know how lucky you are! Imagine, you don't even have to bother with a diaphragm or the pills." She had missed the point entirely. After that I began to realize how difficult it is for fertile people to understand, and I decided to keep my problems to myself.

As the investigation dragged on and my marriage began to wear, the isolation became too much and I sought the help of a psychiatrist, thinking that psychotherapy might help me place the problem in perspective. The young female doctor who saw me had no children, but she seemed understanding. She was the only person who heard about my recurrent nightmare of an empty pram that bounced Eisenstein-like down a vast flight of stairs, always just beyond my reach. The meaning seemed obvious to me. I only hoped that sharing the dream with someone would rid me of it. She pondered long over it and concluded that it clearly showed a deep-rooted conflict between career and children. When she went on to suggest that my infertility might be psychosomatic, she lost my confidence, for even I knew that there were more tests to be performed. I dropped out of therapy and found myself with no one to talk to.

In the course of the whole investigation the most sympathetic understanding — apart from my mother's empathy — came from our friends Anne and Greg, who had been through a similar ordeal. They did not offer unsought medical advice. They did not tell us how lucky we were not to have to worry about birth control. They merely shared with us the feelings they had had during their search. They had felt alone. Their marriage had foundered. They had had erroneous advice. And no one seemed to understand. Worse yet, poor Anne had a mother-in-law who had seemed to call weekly to find out if she was pregnant or not. Just knowing that someone else had somehow gotten through the ordeal was a kind of consolation.

Later, when we finally had a diagnosis and treatment was looming ahead, my closest college friend opened up to me. "Oh Mary," she said, "I have felt so terrible for you. I went through the same thing with my first child. I simply could not bring myself to talk with you because I remember how painful it was for me even to admit I had the problem. And how much I hated interference. I hope everything turns out all right now." As soon as the major part of the anguish was over commiseration came, not only from my college classmate but from many other friends. All had hesitated to bring up the subject, remembering their own pain and isolation.

After they "came out of the closet" I realized how much more help they could have been to me earlier, but I also understood their hesitancy. It has taken me some time to become open about the problem, but I am glad I have, because it makes me available to anyone who wants to talk.

Once, after hearing about the years we had searched in order to have a child, a young woman I had just met stated rather categorically, "But surely you've forgotten all that now."

"No," I replied, "you *never* forget." Two days later she called me to talk about her infertility problem.

The medical community seems to be becoming aware of this aspect of infertility. Infertile couples need to share their problems with people who have similar problems. In certain areas some infertility clinics have initiated meetings for their patients. Elsewhere groups have been formed to provide similar forums for infertile couples. Two such groups are Resolve, Inc. in Massachusetts, and the United Infertility Organization in New York. (See page 170.)

Such groups did not exist when I went through my battle with infertility. They can undoubtedly help, particularly by letting you know you are not alone. If there are no such groups in your community, try to seek out other people who have had a similar problem. Sharing your feelings with other infertile people can help to support you emotionally, and this is important. However, I feel it should be the icing on the cake. Seeking emotional support should go hand in hand with an absolutely thorough investigation of both partners and with the rigorous pursuit of treatments.

PART FOUR

What Treatments Are Available?

After the thorough investigation described in Chapters 7–10, 80 to 95 percent of infertile couples will know what is wrong. In some cases treatment of a minor problem uncovered in the preliminary investigation may begin while the rest of the workup is going on. In other cases diagnosis may not be made until the final test is completed. In some cases a single cause may have been isolated. In other cases more than one problem may have been discovered. Whatever the situation, the correct diagnosis is a major step forward, for then the questions about what constitutes proper treatment for the specific problems can be raised and answered.

It may seem strange to talk of questions when you feel the answer has been found, but the diagnosis, as hard as it may be to make, is but one step. There are numerous questions about treatment, debates about which is the best one for certain problems, arguments about just how successful some of them are. Moreover, the treatments that follow are but other steps on the road toward a successful cure for infertility.

What is considered a cure? What is considered success? The end goal of all treatments is pregnancy carried to term. Yet even the experts are willing to admit that they do not always know exactly how this occurs when it does, or why it sometimes fails to.

My final doctor, who has worked in the field of infertility for over three decades, startled me when I thanked him for helping me become pregnant at last.

"But, Mrs. Harrison, you don't understand," he said. "There is so much we don't know about conception. There are so many variables. All we can do is remove possible hazards so at least there is no obvious impediment to conception. We cannot control the rest. And there is so much still to find out."

The experts do what they can to remove possible hazards, but there is no way they can predict success. In some cases the apparent cause of the infertility can be dealt with, but no pregnancy will follow. In other cases the cause of the infertility may appear to be irresolvable, yet, in rare instances, even without treatment pregnancy will occur. Doctors cannot always explain these phenomena, and they cannot control all the variables.

The treatments available for infertility problems vary in complexity and in the chance of success which they offer. A few problems which are relatively simple have been mentioned earlier, because they are often discovered early in the investigation. Other more complex problems require more complicated treatments. In the female, surgery may be needed to open blocked fallopian tubes, to treat encapsulated ovaries, or to correct malformations of the genital organs. In the male, surgery may be needed for varicocele or other rarer problems. In both male and female, hormonal treatments may be needed to correct an imbalance in the complicated hormonal systems which are involved in the production of germ cells.

If your case is very complicated, you should be willing to seek the help of a specialist. Why do you need a specialist? Because delicate surgery for infertility problems in both men and women requires experienced and skilled hands; even the experts are willing to admit this. In their textbook on female infertility, the late Sophia Kleegman and Sherwin Kaufman report a standard success rate in one surgical procedure to open closed fallopian tubes, but they go on to cite a much higher rate of success for one particular surgeon in Boston.[1] Hormonal treatments for complicated endocrinological problems in women must also be handled by experts who are in daily contact with this relatively new therapy.[2] Some of these treatments require daily surveillance by the physicians and constant checking for adverse side effects.

I balked at first at the idea of seeing a specialist in another city. After all, I thought, the specialists at our university must be as well trained. They were, in fact, but their research centered on a problem I did not have. So I traveled to another city to receive a correct diagnosis and then surgery from an expert. I was not alone. In the course of my treatment, I met women in the doctor's waiting room who had traveled from all over the United States, and even from Europe and South America.

Just as the treatments vary, so also do the rates of success measured in terms of subsequent pregnancies. None of the treatments offers a 100 percent guarantee of pregnancy. However, to an infertile couple with no chance of conceiving without surgery or complicated hormonal therapy, even a 15 percent chance of success seems large. I did not even inquire about the chance of pregnancy. Without surgery, we had no chance.

Treatments for the Woman

THE TREATMENTS for female problems vary according to the problem uncovered. The discussion that follows will be divided according to the sites of possible problems.

The Vagina and Cervix

Congenital anomalies or malformations of the vagina and cervix, and local growths in either area, are physical impediments to conception and are usually treated surgically. The most commonly found growths are cervical polyps, bits of tissue which block the opening of the cervix and prevent the passage of sperm. These are usually excised, but great care must be taken to cut as conservatively as possible in order not to damage the tissue of the cervix that produces the secretions favorable to sperm at the time of ovulation. Congenital anomalies of the vagina and cervix are extremely rare, but they too can sometimes be treated surgically. If all other pelvic organs are normal and functioning correctly, the surgical correction of these physical problems can result in pregnancy in some cases.

Infections or inflammations of the vagina and cervix inhibit conception because they create secretions which are inimical to sperm, preventing viable sperm from reaching the egg. These infections or inflammations can be treated with drugs, as are other infections of the body, or with local application of silver nitrate. Both of these are relatively simple therapies, and minor infections respond well to them. Many gynecologists routinely use electrocauterization, a technique in which infections or areas of inflammation are burned off. However, infertility specialists advise extreme caution in use of this technique. If the cauterization burns too deeply or extensively, the tissue of the cervix that produces secretions favorable to sperm at the time of ovulation may be permanently damaged. For the same reason, most specialists are adamantly opposed to conization, the surgical removal of the infected or inflamed part of the cervix, for this may alter even more radically the tissue of the cervix and its secretions.[1]

Some women have problems with "hostile" cervical mucus. Rather than producing a secretion favorable to sperm penetration and migration at the time of ovulation, the cervix of these women produces acid secretions which inhibit the progress of sperm. Some experts attempt to change the character of the mucus by prescribing a daily dosage of a very small amount of synthetic estrogen.[2] In an occasional case, doctors may recommend an alkaline douche immediately before intercourse during the fertile period to make the vagina and mucus more receptive to sperm by altering the acidity.[3]

The Uterus

Congenital malformations of the uterus vary in type and may be discovered as a cause of repeated miscarriages. They show up clearly on hysterosalpingography. These malformations are rare, but when they are encountered, surgery may be the treatment of choice. One malformation which can cause miscarriage is bicornuate uterus, in which the upper part of the uterus is divided into two hornlike projections. In this case, the surgeon attempts to correct the situation by reconstructing a normal upper part of the uterus so that the uterus can expand to contain a growing fetus.

Fibroid tumors, benign fibrous growths in the uterine wall, are often found in women in their thirties. If they are severe in size or number, they can prevent implantation of a fertilized egg. You should know that many gynecologists standardly recommend a hysterectomy for this condition. If your doctor advises hysterectomy and you want to have children, you should get a second opinion. Infertility specialists stress that surgical removal of the tumors is possible, in an operation called a myomectomy.[4] This operation removes only the tumors and leaves the uterus intact for future childbearing. Doctors who are anxious to preserve the childbearing function of any woman who desires it might recommend myomectomy before resorting to the more drastic measure of hysterectomy. However, before undertaking myomectomy, the doctor must rule out all other possible causes of infertility.

Different surgeons report success rates as between 30 and 60 percent following myomectomy, but they stress the importance of early action.[5] The chances of success diminish as the patient ages and as the fibroids proliferate and grow. Two experts remark upon the occasional necessity for more than one operation, citing a case of a woman who underwent two myomectomies before finally conceiving and bearing a child.[6] When pregnancy ensues following this kind of operation, delivery by a caesarean section is often recommended.

Diseases of the endometrium, the lining of the uterus, can cause adhesions and can impede the implantation of a fertilized egg. These diseases may be discovered on endometrial biopsy, but specialists warn that they may go undetected if the biopsy does not include an adequate amount of tissue from high up in the body of the uterus.[7] For this reason, some experts recommend that several samples of tissue be taken from different locations in the uterus in an endometrial biopsy.[8] If infections are discovered, antibiotics can be used; but specialists urge further tests as well, since an infection of the endometrium may be associated with infections of the tubes that could cause tubal blockages. What can be done about these adhesions? The answer depends on the severity of the condition. In some cases adhesions caused by endometrial diseases can be removed with conservative surgery.

The Fallopian Tubes

The problems most commonly discovered in the fallopian tubes are those that prevent the meeting of egg and sperm — either complete or partial blockage of the tubes or peritubal adhesions that interfere with the mobility of the tubes. These conditions can be the result of a variety of different problems, as discussed in Chapters 3 and 7. Moreover, the conditions vary in their location within the fallopian tube, in their severity, and in the kinds of treatment they seem to warrant.

In some cases medical treatment of the problem appears to be called for. There are two general types of medical treatment, both using the same kind of apparatus used in the Rubin test for tubal insufflation. One involves repeated insufflation of the tubes with carbon dioxide, a procedure that may succeed in opening minor blockages or straightening out kinked tubes. The other involves infusion of the tubes with a special medicine in an attempt to clear up minor infections and open the tubes at the same time.

In other cases surgery may be called for. Many gynecologists, however, are discouraged by poor results reported in the medical literature and may advise against this kind of surgery. One of my doctors did. But since some success is reported for all of these surgical procedures, the infertile couple may wish to go through with an operation.

Nevertheless, it is extremely important to seek an expert. One such expert, Celso-Ramon Garcia of the University of Pennsylvania in Philadelphia, has written that "many surgeons view the surgical treatment of the oviduct [fallopian tubes] in the infertile patient as being very simple in comparison to other forms of abdominal pelvic surgery." [9] Dr. Garcia goes on to stress that this kind of surgery is, in fact, very "exacting."

Surgeons experienced in reconstructing the oviduct should be sought.

However, before proceeding to surgery all other possible causes of infertility must be ruled out. All pelvic inflammatory disease (PID) must be ruled out or cleared up by treatment. In some cases doctors may even try preliminary medical treatment of the type described above before moving on to surgery. Most important, tubal blockages should be confirmed by hysterosalpingography.[10] In this way the doctor can pinpoint the location of the blockages and decide how to proceed. If blockages are found at both ends of the tubes, the prognosis is extremely poor.[11] Blockages in other areas may be operated on with some degree of success in a certain percentage of cases.

Operations on the fallopian tubes vary according to the area of the tube which is involved. Blockages may exist either at the fundal end, where the tubes attach to the uterus, or in the midsection. The outer ends of the tubes may also be totally or partially closed.

The most favorable results have been reported for operations on the outer ends of tubes that are only partially blocked. In fimbriolysis, the doctor enlarges the already existing opening of the tube by separating the fimbriae that may be stuck together. In salpingolysis, he attempts to remove peritubal adhesions around the opening. Some doctors report a success rate of 35 to 40 percent with these procedures.[12]

Operations for blockages at midsection and at the fundal end of the tubes seem to have slightly less favorable results, although success rates as high as 35 to 40 percent have been reported by certain doctors.[13] In these procedures the blocked areas of the tubes are excised and then the clean ends of the tubes are joined. In the operation on the fundal end, some surgeons advise the use of a splint to keep the tube open.

The least favorable results have been reported for salpingoplasty, an operation to correct complete blockages of the outer end of the tubes. In this operation doctors must create an entirely new tubal opening. The difficulties of this kind of surgery are enormous, for not only does the tube have to remain open after surgery, it also has to acquire or reacquire its normal physiological function. Some doctors insert a silastic hood in a first operation to keep the tube open, with removal of the hood to follow in a second operation some time later.[14] Other doctors are not so convinced that the hood is absolutely necessary.[15] In spite of the obvious complexities of this kind of surgery, some pregnancies have been reported, but only in 15 to 25 percent of cases.[16]

All of these operations can result in reestablishing patency of the tubes in a certain percentage of cases. However, in order for pregnancy to occur, full physiological functioning of the tubes must also return so that the tube can capture the egg and succeed in transporting it to the uterus, and surgery cannot insure this.

Irresolvable blockage of the tubes is one of the most frustrating diagnoses, because the woman knows she is producing an egg which simply does not have the path on which to travel to meet the sperm. Experiments are going on now to try to solve this discouraging problem, and they will be described in Chapter 20. To date, the medical and surgical treatments described above are the treatments most generally available for specific problems of the fallopian tubes.

The Ovaries

Ovaries with multiple cysts, also called polycystic ovaries, can cause infertility in some cases. When the cysts are associated with symptoms such as the absence of menstruation, enlarged ovaries, excessive hair growth, and occasionally obesity, a diagnosis of Stein-Leventhal syndrome can be made. But the cysts can be present in the ovaries without causing any of the above symptoms, so a careful diagnosis should be made. The cysts may represent the failure of the ovaries to release eggs, so this condition must be treated.

The physician may first try to induce ovulation and effect the release of eggs by administering drugs affecting the adrenal glands or with drugs affecting the ovaries. If these drugs do not succeed in reestablishing ovulation or if the disease seems very advanced, the doctor may choose to perform a surgical procedure known as a wedge resection. In this procedure a triangular piece, like a wedge of melon, is cut out of the ovary and then the ovary is sewed up. Experts do not fully understand how this procedure succeeds in reestablishing ovulation, but it does in a large percentage of cases. Some doctors have reported that ovulation can return in 80 to 90 percent of cases, with pregnancy in as many as 60 percent of cases. [17]

Pelvic Diseases

Many diseases can affect any or all of the pelvic organs to prevent conception, and they require varying treatments.

Acute pelvic inflammatory disease or PID is a general name for acute inflammations or infections of the pelvic organs. According to Richard H. Schwarz, Professor of Obstetrics and Gynecology at the University of Pennsylvania, gonorrhea accounts for 60 percent of all diagnosed cases of PID. [18] Infections caused by other organisms or by peritonitis following a ruptured appendix are less commonly found. These diseases are not always associated with infertility, but in their advanced stages, they can block or damage the fallopian tubes and seriously affect fertility.

Acute pelvic inflammatory disease is widespread in the United States. Gonorrhea is on the rise and it may be that this will lead to increased problems with infertility in the future. Because of its prevalence and its serious nature, the problem of pelvic inflammatory disease will be described fully.

Gonorrhea, a venereal disease affecting both men and women, poses problems of diagnosis. In its early stages in women, when it is present in the lower genital tract, it can be very hard to diagnose. The symptoms may be very mild, or there may be no symptoms at all. Dr. Schwarz has estimated that the disease is asymptomatic in as many as nine out of ten cases in women.[19] If the disease goes untreated or is not treated sufficiently, it can spread to the upper genital tract where it can cause serious damage to the fallopian tubes. It can be associated with blockages or closure of the tubes; it can also be involved in limiting tubal mobility.

Gonorrhea must first be treated vigorously with antibiotics until a cure is achieved. If the fallopian tubes have been affected, surgery may then be required. However, if the disease is very advanced or if the tubes are extensively damaged, there is not much hope for subsequent pregnancy.

Tuberculosis of the genital organs or pelvis is another cause of infertility, but it is found only rarely in the United States. It does occur more frequently in areas of the world where there is a higher incidence of pulmonary tuberculosis.[20]

Like PID, tuberculosis can be present with no symptoms other than infertility, so diagnosis must be made carefully. Like PID, tuberculosis usually causes infertility by affecting the tubes. Very advanced cases have the poorest prognosis of all causes of infertility, for even if the tuberculosis can be cured, the tubes may be irreparably damaged.

Endometriosis is an enigmatic disease in which endometrial tissue is extruded or appears outside the uterus. This tissue implants in various sites and responds to female hormones, waxing, waning, and bleeding in accordance with the menstrual cycle. It can cause infertility by implanting on the ovaries and preventing the release of the egg, by interfering with the tubal pickup of the egg, by blocking the openings of the tubes, or by adhering to the tubes and interfering with their mobility. The disease is often difficult to diagnose, for, like tuberculosis, it can be present with no symptoms other than infertility. In my case it was discovered only on culdoscopy.

Experts are divided on the cause of the disease.[21] Some maintain that the tissue is extruded through the tubes into the peritoneum during menstruation. For this reason, experts oppose tubal insufflation during menstruation.[22] Others feel that the tissue can arise spontaneously in the abdomen. Whatever the cause, the disease is more common in women who have delayed childbearing, and it seems to improve when ovulation is suppressed.

On learning of my condition, a friend of mine who had had endometriosis commiserated and then said, "You know there is a dreadful psychological profile for people with endometriosis. We're well educated, in our late twenties, usually white, and we're overanxious, egocentric, and perfectionist." I laughed nervously as I recognized myself in her description, and I dismissed the idea until I read the same profile in a comprehensive article on the disease.[23] Then I began to ponder it in light of my experience with the disease.

Did I fit the stereotype of the patient with endometriosis? If so, what did the stereotype mean? Well educated and in my late twenties? Yes, I had earned the Ph.D. degree and had put off having children to do it. My age alone was one answer to why I had endometriosis. Overanxious and perfectionist? Yes, but what did that mean? That anxiety caused the disease? I was not convinced, but I was certain that, had I not been overanxious and perfectionist, I never would have pursued the diagnosis as I had done. Egocentric? Certainly. But that meant that I cared about my body and its proper functioning — again, a reason to pursue the diagnosis for three long years. The profile may be accurate for those who insist on finding out what is wrong. But I wonder how many unselfish and underanxious women there are with endometriosis. They may have "silent" cases, which remain undiagnosed because their first doctors tell them nothing is wrong and they do not push for an answer as I did.

Endometriosis exists in some cases with no symptoms other than infertility, but in other cases there are various symptoms. The most common one is extreme pain at the time of menstruation. Other symptoms are pain on intercourse, pain on urinating or defecating, blood in the urine, or a diminished menstrual flow. However, these general symptoms do not always indicate that endometriosis is present, so a careful diagnosis is necessary.

Endometriosis may be treated in different ways, depending on its severity. Women with minor symptoms and only a minimal amount of endometriosis visible on culdoscopy or laparoscopy may be observed for a time and given analgesics to control pain. More extensive endometriosis can be treated in two ways. First, the doctor may choose to suppress ovulation with hormones. The patient takes high doses of hormonal preparations, such as birth control pills, continuously for several months, to prevent ovulation and menstruation. If the patient does not menstruate, then the bits of endometrial tissue inside will not grow and bleed either. They may even diminish, and this is the desired end of treatment. A second treatment is surgery for cases in which endometriosis is extensive or has caused significant adhesions. In my case, the endometriosis was so widespread that it had engulfed the ovaries in a hard shell and formed so many adhesions on the tubes that it almost totally joined the fimbriae of one tube and interfered drastically with the mobility of both tubes. The surgeon excised areas of endometrial tissue, and he also performed a wedge resection on the ovaries and fimbriolysis on one of the tubes. Experts urge very conservative and cautious surgery in order to preserve the childbearing capacities as much as possible. Surgery may be followed by a course of hormone therapy to suppress ovulation. Surgeons have reported a 30 to 40 percent rate of success in these operations.

As is the case with so many difficulties described in this book, endometriosis requires the opinion of infertility experts. One of my friends was told that the only certain cure for her endometriosis was hysterectomy. The advice was sound enough, since hysterectomy is the only way to eliminate the disease completely. But a woman who is seeking a cure to enable her to have children does not want to hear advice that would end her search forever. Experts in infertility, who often encounter situations like my friend's, urge caution. Robert J. Kistner, Clinical Professor of Obstetrics and Gynecology at the Harvard Medical School, has written: "Pregnancies have been noted subsequent to treatment in patients to whom hysterectomy had been suggested." [24]

Indeed, whenever any woman is advised to have a hysterectomy before she has had children or completed her family, she should seek a second opinion. Many conditions for which hysterectomy is sometimes recommended, like endometriosis or fibroid tumors, can respond to more conservative treatment. A more conservative approach preserves at least the possibility of childbearing, a possibility that vanishes once a hysterectomy is performed.

Hormonal Problems

Disorders of the thyroid and adrenal glands can cause infertility. Hypothyroidism, the underfunctioning of the thyroid gland, may show up in preliminary lab tests and can be treated with thyroid medication. This therapy can cure the specific malfunction of the thyroid gland so that the normal functioning of the entire female hormonal system can resume. Adrenogenital syndrome is a complicated malfunctioning of the adrenal glands that affects the activity of the pituitary gland. This syndrome must be carefully diagnosed; it can be treated with cortisone with varying degrees of success.

More commonly encountered endocrinological problems of the female involve the hypothalamic-pituitary-ovarian network described on pages 17–18. When there are disturbances in this network of glands, ovulation may not occur at all or it may occur so rarely that conception is highly unlikely. Problems with ovulation may be discovered before an infertility workup because the patient fails to menstruate. However, because a woman can menstruate without ovulating, she may discover problems with ovulation only when she fails to become pregnant. In an infertility investigation the presence of these problems may be indicated by the Basal Body Temperature Charts, endometrial biopsy, or more complex endocrinological studies such as the analysis of hormone excretion in a twenty-four-hour collection of urine. It is important to stress that anovulation, the cessation of ovulation, can be associated with other medical problems and that these should be ruled out or corrected at the outset. In a majority of cases, however, these medical problems are not at work.

In the past very little could be done about anovulation that was unrelated to medical disorders. As late as the early fifties doctors were attempting to treat anovulation by irradiating the pituitary or the ovaries with X ray. This procedure did not have much success, and it was risky because of the harmful effects of radiation. Wedge resection, one of the surgical procedures described on page 102, has also been used — and continues to be used — to treat anovulation. Even though doctors do not understand exactly how this procedure works, it can restore ovulation in certain cases.

Since the late fifties, however, new methods for treating anovulation have been developed. These involve the use of drugs or hormonal preparations.[25]

Clomiphene citrate, a drug known as Clomid, appears to work best on women who ovulate infrequently and who produce small amounts of the pituitary messengers, FSH and LH. Taken in tablet form, Clomid seems to work by activating or promoting the production of pituitary hormones, which can then work on the ovaries to stimulate ovulation. When infertility is solely the result of infrequent production of eggs, Clomid can result in ovulation in 70 to 80 percent of cases and in pregnancy in about 40 to 50 percent of cases.[26] Greater knowledge about dosages has decreased the side effects that were present when the drug was first introduced, but some of these still can occur. Ovarian cysts, the result of the stimulation of numerous follicles, are one side effect, but they are usually only temporary. Multiple births can occur following Clomid therapy; twins are reported in about 10 percent of cases.[27] Finally, even after one pregnancy, a woman may return to an anovulatory state and may need Clomid again if she wants another child.

Another preparation, Pergonal or human menopausal gonadotropin (HMG), may be used in women who do not ovulate and who do not appear to produce any pituitary messengers. This preparation consists of actual pituitary hormones extracted from the urine of postmenopausal women and then purified. It must be administered by injection because it is not effective in tablet form. In effect, it is a substitute for the woman's own pituitary messenger, FSH, and it is used to try to stimulate the ovaries to produce eggs. It must be administered sequentially with a second hormonal preparation which acts like LH. This second preparation is injected to stimulate the release of the egg at the appropriate moment in the woman's cycle. The dosages must be very carefully regulated, as there is an extremely fine line between the amount of Pergonal necessary to stimulate the growth of an egg and the amount which results in overstimulated ovaries. When properly administered, the drug can result in ovulation in 90 percent of the cases and in pregnancy in 50 to 70 percent of cases.[28] The incidence of multiple births with Pergonal is higher than with Clomid, occurring in 20 percent of cases.[29]

Not all patients with hormonal upsets are candidates for these modes of therapy. Cases must be carefully screened beforehand and carefully followed during treatment. All other possible physical problems and causes of infertility must be ruled out. The existence of ovarian response must be proven. Before initiating therapy, the doctor must have a clear idea of the state of the patient's pelvis and the nature of the patient's temperature charts, in order to be able to judge any changes that occur after treatment. Drs. Speroff, Glass, and Kase of Yale University describe the complexities of this therapy and stress that an endocrinological expert must evaluate and follow these cases.

In both therapies, the patient and her husband must follow exactly the regimen prescribed. There is a rigid timetable for the administration of the drugs. Basal Body Temperature Charts must be scrupulously accurate. Scheduled intercourse will be demanded. Frequent visits to the physician may be necessary to check for adverse side effects. Both therapies are costly (although Clomid is considerably less expensive than Pergonal), and both are short term, efficacious only in the one cycle in which they are administered.

Immunological Problems

Immunological factors have been recently discovered as another possible cause of infertility, and research is being conducted in this area.[30] One specific immunologic condition has been defined and treatment has been developed. In this condition, a wife is allergic to her husband's sperm and her body develops antibodies which immobilize his sperm in her body. Laboratory testing can uncover the problem, and the recommended treatment is relatively simple. The wife must avoid all contact with her husband's sperm for several months — no oral-genital sex and the use of condoms at all times. At the end of six months, the woman should be retested for the allergy. If she is still allergic, condom therapy can continue. If she is no longer allergic, the couple can try to conceive. Pregnancies have been reported following this therapy.

The most frustrating diagnosis after a thorough infertility workup is undiagnosed infertility. Some experts find this in 20 percent of their cases, while others find it in only 5 percent. According to a study by Anna Southam of Columbia University a certain percentage of these couples may conceive after several years of infertility.[31] For the others, the only hope that can be offered is that continuing research in the field may uncover new causes and new methods of treatment. Ten years ago, couples with immunological problems undoubtedly were assessed as cases of undiagnosed infertility; but today it is possible to identify their problem and to treat it. Tomorrow still other causes and treatments may be found.

CHAPTER 13

Treatment: A Personal View

THE COMPLICATED treatments for the complex causes of female infertility have been described in Chapter 12. However, the mere enumeration of treatments available cannot convey the continual anxieties the patient feels as she undergoes treatment. The experts understand thoroughly the complexities and risks of the various therapies. They see your therapy with eyes that have seen hundreds of other cases. You as a patient, however, are likely to view the problem differently. You see but one problem, your own, and one goal, a future pregnancy. What, then, is treatment like for a patient? I cannot generalize here, because your treatment may be different from mine, your reactions may vary. So the two accounts which follow will simply present the way I felt during my own treatment and the way I viewed the experience of a friend of mine.

Surgery: A Personal Experience

For my husband and me, the most frustrating part of infertility was the long journey to diagnosis. So many years had gone by searching for what was wrong. Our marriage had reeled with every bit of bad news the earlier tests had brought. We had often encountered tenative diagnoses which turned out to be erroneous. The gynecologist's assertions that the sperm count was too low had assailed my husband's ego. My conviction that my tubes were hopelessly closed had struck at my self-confidence. Yet the marriage had survived, stronger than before, as we both came to realize that our world would not end without children. Nonetheless we had persisted until we finally had the diagnosis. Once we had that, we knew definitely what treatment would follow.

Our specialist, who was a man of few words, met with us after my culdoscopy. "Well, we finally have a diagnosis," he said. "It's not that we know anything more than doctors in other cities. We just like to be thorough, to get a good history, to do all the tests possible."

He then asked us matter-of-factly when we wanted to schedule surgery. "How about June?" he said.

I nodded assent. I would have agreed if he'd said tomorrow.

"Could we schedule it before my husband goes off to a conference in Europe?" I inquired politely.

"In Europe? Were you planning to go with him? We can do the operation in July just as well. After three years, one month won't make that much difference. It just has to be timed before you ovulate."

So we counted ahead, estimated the ovulation date, and reserved a room in the hospital for July.

My admiration for the doctor was — and still is — boundless. He was a thorough physician. He had carefully looked over my temperature charts; he was the first one to tell me he was looking for luteal phase deficiencies as well as for evidence of ovulation. He had asked to see the X rays of the hysterosalpinogram for himself. He also was not overly concerned that my husband's sperm count was in the lower ranges of normal. "Twenty million is low, but perfectly adequate. Why, I know an obstetrician with that count who has had five children." He also was the first one to make a correct diagnosis of my condition. It was no wonder I had absolute trust in his judgment. Once we had found him, we were ready to do whatever he suggested.

When he told us surgery was needed, I did not inquire about the success rate for my operation. I did not ask what were the chances I'd get pregnant. I had to be operated on. Given that fact, my chief concern was what kind of scar the doctor would give me. When I asked him, he asserted that a midline incision would give him greater visibility. So I resigned myself to giving up my bikinis. If he wanted a midline incision, he could have it. He knew what he needed. He told me, though, to remind him to use subcutaneous stitches.

"What kind of stitches?" I asked my husband after we'd left the office.

"Subcutaneous, under the skin," he answered and explained that these were stitches in the next-to-last layer of skin that made less of a scar.

Only after the operation was over did my husband tell me how much he had worried about the risks of surgery. He was supremely confident in the doctor's abilities. But as a physician he had seen enough surgery to know all the things that could go wrong. In any major operation one could encounter problems with adverse reactions to anesthesia, unsuspected problems with the procedure itself, and so forth. He did not want to alarm me, so he worried in silence and only revealed his anxiety once, when he advised me in a half-joking manner to paint my name across my abdomen.

"I don't want them mixing you up with another patient and performing a hysterectomy on you," he said.

I laughed uneasily and thought seriously about taking an indelible pen with me to the hospital.

However, I tried not to worry unduly, and as my working year came to an end, I prepared to enjoy Europe as I never had before. I fell in love again with the red palaces of Rome, savored the smells of horses and garlic, listened with renewed delight to the splash of water in the fountains, and ate pasta to my heart's content, knowing I would lose weight after surgery.

The last night in Rome, we went to the Trevi fountain. I threw in two coins — one for my husband and me and one for the baby I hoped we would have. But if there's no baby, I reminded myself realistically, then those two coins are for two more trips to Rome. We'll do all we can to get that baby but if no baby comes, we'll still have a full life.

Time flew by, and suddenly I was in the hospital. I almost looked forward to the operation. I willingly took all the pills and shots they gave me to make me drowsy before surgery. Alternately dozing and awaking as I waited for the orderly, I kept reminding myself, "Make sure the doctor knows who you are and don't forget subcutaneous, subcutaneous."

When the orderly finally came, she apologized for the delay — needlessly, because I had lost all track of time. But I tried to stir myself as she wheeled me to the operating room.

My doctor smiled as he saw me coming and greeted me, repeating my name to assure me I was in the right operating room.

I remember that I was so dazed by the medication that I had difficulty pronouncing his name. But somehow I was able to ask clear as day, "Remember to give me subcutaneous stitches."

He looked somewhat startled. "Why? Do you have other scars?"

"No," I managed to answer. "But I like bikinis." And I dozed off again.

When I awoke after surgery, I was aware only of sunlight, searing pain, and striped curtains. The nurses were quick to give me more medication when I asked for it. And later that day, my husband gently fed me ice chips as he repeated to me what the doctor had told him over the telephone.

"It *was* endometriosis. *Everywhere* apparently. Yes, he cleaned it up. He took out your appendix too. Thought you had had appendicitis before. It's all right. Yes, it's all right," he told me again and again.

The same orderly who had taken me to the operating room

transferred me back to my regular bed. "You were the calmest patient I've ever seen," she remarked. "I nearly flipped when you asked for subcutaneous stitches."

Her good humor gave me strength, but it was a few days before I actually looked at the bandage. I could not resist a smile when I saw a "bikini scar," straight across my lower abdomen.

I was in the hospital a week, gaining strength daily and not losing as much weight as I had thought I would. I slept a lot, read, and made lists of questions to ask the doctor. He answered some of them laconically, but he never chatted for very long. I remarked on this to my husband when he came to visit.

"He's a busy man," he reminded me. "Which would you rather have? Someone who holds your hand and does not make the diagnosis? Or expert treatment?"

My roommate overheard our conversation and jumped in to agree with my husband. "He is quiet. But he's a master." She was recovering from her third operation. The first two had brought her a baby girl. Now she was trying for a second child.

She had told me all about her experience. It was similar to ours — years of investigation, and finally treatment away from home. Two operations, before pregnancy! And even after the operations, her pregnancy had not been easy. Now she was having problems conceiving again.

When she had threatened to miscarry in the sixth month of that first pregnancy, the doctor put her in the hospital, flat on her back, for the remaining three months. "Once the doctor succeeds in getting you pregnant," she said, "he'll do everything in the world to get that baby here." Her case gave me hope: she had gotten pregnant. But she also made me see that a single operation did not guarantee anything.

It took me six weeks to the day, as the doctor had predicted, to regain full strength. Occasionally I had bursts of energy in the morning which would fizzle out by eleven. I remember lots of rest and endless hours of Watergate. They had shot for the moon in 1969 and in 1973 their target was the president. The "gavel to gavel coverage" was a godsend, though, and I became attuned to every twitch of Senator Ervin's eyebrows.

The surgery was followed by a three-month course of hormones to create a pseudopregnancy and to forestall any further growth of endometriosis. I had hoped for a real pregnancy, but I had to be content with a fake one for three months. I did not like the idea of taking birth control pills. I had never used them as a contraceptive. I was dismayed at the seventeen pounds I gained. And I became very worried when my legs began to ache. Was I developing thrombosis? I was examined by the doctor and was told not to worry. I tried, not very successfully. And I kept reminding myself that there were just a few weeks left of the three-month period. Then, maybe, just maybe, pregnancy would follow.

When I stopped taking the pills, all the anxieties we had had before returned. But it was worse this time. If I couldn't get pregnant after surgery, we had come to the end of the road. Temperature charts in the morning, programmed intercourse every other night, and baited breath at the end of each cycle. Two months later, five and a half months after the operation, I began to resign myself once again to a life without children.

"Look, we've done all we can," my husband said. "You had to have the operation anyway, for your own health. We'll make a good life for ourselves."

So we planned a spring trip to New York City. I received the two-year teaching contract I had been hoping for. And when we went to New York, I got my hair cut for the first time in seven years, treating myself to a special beauty day at a fancy hair salon.

Two months later, I despaired once again when a twinge of premenstrual cramping announced yet another failure. But incredibly, no menstruation followed. I was scared to have a pregnancy test, scared that just taking the urine sample into the lab would jinx us somehow. But my husband insisted, and I let him go to the lab alone. That afternoon, he returned waving a lab slip in my face. It read simply: "Physician's wife. Preg Pos."

The temperature chart told us the exact moment of conception. It was eight and a half months after the operation, and one month to the day after I had had my hair cut.

Caroline's Case History

My friend Caroline had had an experience similar to ours in searching for a diagnosis. She had been told that she was "normal" and her husband's low sperm count had been blamed. But she, too, had felt intuitively that something was wrong with her.

"Listen, Mary, my temperature charts are really irregular. I can't see a definite swing upward. Something *must* be wrong," she insisted during one of our frequent phone calls. We had discovered each other as confidantes in a doctor's waiting room and our long hours of conversation there had led to friendship. Our problem linked us together, too, so we commiserated and shared information on a regular basis.

At her insistence, the doctor referred her to specialists at the university nearby. Several months later, her problem had been isolated: pituitary insufficiency. Her pituitary gland did not send out the right message of FSH each month. Her ovaries therefore received inadequate stimulus to produce eggs regularly.

She tried to look on the light side when she told me. "You'll never believe this, but, dammit, my mother was right. It *must* be all in my head — it's my pituitary."

We had complained bitterly to each other about the unsought-for advice each of us received from well-meaning people. I had comforted her when her mother screamed at her that it was "all in her head." And she had solaced me when my friend Gay had told me how lucky I was not to have to use birth control. At least we two knew how hard it was for others to understand.

"Your pituitary?" How did they find out?" I queried. And she told me about the new interpretations of the temperature charts and the results of the tests on her twenty-four-hour urine sample.

"What can they do?" I asked.

"Well, you know, we're really lucky. There's a drug, Clomid, that's supposed to act on the pituitary. They're going to try it on me, starting next month."

So her experience with Clomid began. But in spite of her high hopes, there was no immediate change in her temperature charts or on other tests. After three months of failure, the dosage was increased, but still there were no positive results. Every morning she held the thermometer in her mouth longer than the usual five minutes, hoping for some rise. Even the slightest change produced wonder and fears. She nursed fears of ovarian enlargement in silence. Finally, after many months had gone by, the maximum dosage had failed to stimulate ovulation, and the doctors ground to a halt.

"What am I going to do?" she wailed. "They are taking me off Clomid. They've talked about an experimental drug, Pergonal. And they are one of the few places in the country that can give it. But I'm not sure I want to be used as a guinea pig. There is danger of overstimulated ovaries. And multiple births too."

But after long discussions with her husband, she decided that they had no chance otherwise. So her treatment with Pergonal began. Her husband learned how to give her injections and they braced themselves for the cost. The first month, she called me almost every day.

This treatment seems to me now to have been even more demanding than ours later turned out to be. She described the horrors of her husband giving her shots every night. And every morning careful recordings of her temperature and her weight. The idea of making love was almost a nightmare to them; and yet, they knew that programmed intercourse was in store for them. The doctors demanded to see her every day to palpate her ovaries, to check the temperature and weight charts, and to look for changes in the cervical mucus, changes which would indicate the stimulation of hormonal activity. They ordered her once again to collect all her urine output over a twenty-four-hour period. She had done this before when they were checking out her hormonal system. Now it seemed even more crucial, for it would establish whether the estrogen level was rising.

Then one day she called me, exultant. "The cervical mucus has changed, and the estrogen level is up. They gave me a shot of HCG (human chorionic gonadotropin) this morning. We're supposed to have intercourse tonight and again in two days. But then, nothing. The ovaries may be so stimulated that they are too fragile for any other intense physical activity. What have we gotten into?"

She was fearful of what she was doing to her body, afraid that with this experimental drug she might in some way damage herself. She wanted desperately to have a child, but she was frightened at the possibility of twins, or triplets — or even more.

When she became pregnant in the following month, she crowed and I shared her excitement. But I also shared her anxious months of not knowing how many babies she had conceived. And as I saw her anxiety, I realized that no one — not even her husband — could feel what she was feeling, a dread that did not disperse until she found out that only one child was on its way.

She had conceived, and she bore a child. But when she and her husband decided they wanted to try to have another child, the same process had to be repeated. And the same apprehensions returned. Now, with two healthy children, she can look back on the experience with some degree of equanimity, recognizing that before the discovery of Pergonal in the late fifties, women with her problem had no hope of children.

CHAPTER 14

Treatments for the Man

THE MEN with infertility problems are in a more difficult situation than many women are. For one thing, no absolutely successful hormonal treatment for azoospermia or extreme oligospermia, the absence of sperm or an extremely low number of sperm, has been discovered to date, in contrast to the recent developments in hormonal treatment of ovulatory failure in women. For another, there is a larger gray area in male infertility, the frustrating diagnosis of the borderline sperm count, which may or may not be responsible for a couple's infertility and may or may not improve with simple health measures. No absolutely efficacious treatment has yet been found for the borderline sperm count. In fact, the causes of male infertility that can be treated with a reasonable degree of success are few in number. And there is another problem: the diagnosis of a borderline or poor sperm count can lead doctors to stop investigating the female and thus to overlook a "silent" and causative factor in the woman, as happened in our case. Work is being done on male problems, so there is hope for future developments. But what is the situation at present? What are the problems? What treatments are available?

The conditions that seem very problematic and untreatable in most instances are azoospermia or extreme oligospermia, Equally problematic are the conditions in which a very high percentage or all of the sperm are immobile or abnormally shaped. However, when these diagnoses are first made, you should not immediately give up the investigation, because these conditions may be caused by temporary factors, such as recent illness.

A borderline sperm count is an even bigger question mark. Such a count may often be cited as a possible cause of infertility, as it was in our case. The most frustrating part about this diagnosis is its vagueness, for the term *borderline* can describe counts that range as widely as from ten to forty million sperm per milliliter with slightly less than standard percentages of motile and normally shaped sperm. Pregnancy is not totally ruled out, but it may be declared to be highly unlikely. In these cases, however, there is always a chance. It seems worth repeating John MacLeod's advice to complete the investigation of the female when a borderline count is in question, because he has seen ". . . pregnancies . . . occur in the chronic presence of appalling semen quality." [1]

The treatment for a borderline sperm count may seem as vague to the patient as the definition. Most doctors continue to advise rest, daily exercise, a balanced diet, vitamins, limited consumption of alcohol and tobacco, and improvement of general health. In addition, physicians counsel that the patient should be careful to avoid exposing the genitals to heat. The patient with oligospermia should avoid long hot baths, tight underpants, and even the regular prolonged periods of sitting that some jobs necessitate. Finally, some doctors advise that men with oligospermia avoid taking any drugs or medication whatsoever, since recent research has shown that some groups of drugs can adversely affect the production of sperm. [2]

Many experts feel that this kind of advice is probably most helpful for men whose sperm counts are in the low range of twenty to forty million sperm per milliliter. [3] Others feel that the efficacy of these measures has yet to be proved scientifically. However, Dr. Melvin Taymor of the Harvard Medical School writes convincingly that "if one holds to the concept that improving male fertility to any degree whatsoever is helpful to the female partner, there is every reason to pursue this course regardless of our present inability to prove statistical significance." [4]

You may feel that all these measures seem like only general advice for good health. Are there no treatments to improve spermatogenesis in men, you may wonder, that are comparable to the hormonal treatments recently developed to improve ovulation in women?

The Question of Drug Therapy

Various hormonal treatments to improve sperm count have been tried — and continue to be experimented with — but none has had the resounding success that comparable treatments for women have had.

Specific drug therapy is warranted when endocrine dysfunction is diagnosed in laboratory tests. Patients with diagnosed pituitary problems have been treated with human chorionic gonadotropin (HCG) in combination with human menopausal gonadotropin (HMG), and some success has been reported. Diagnosed dysfunctions of the thyroid and adrenal glands can be treated and cured in most cases with appropriate medications.

Nonspecific drug therapy for oligospermia has been advocated by some physicians even when no definable endocrine dysfunction can be diagnosed. They argue that since some positive results have been reported with these therapies, they may be helpful for reasons that are still not clearly understood medically. [5]

Thyroid medication (Cytomel) has been used to augment or stimulate the activity of the thyroid gland in an effort to improve its functioning, particularly in its relationships with the glands involved in spermatogenesis. Opinion is divided on its use, however. Doctors Speroff, Kase, and Glass of Yale University are particularly strongly opposed to using this medication if there is no definable problem with the thyroid gland. [6] Dr. Bruce Stewart feels that an unwarranted use of thyroid medication may actually lower an already low count.[7] Others feel that a small dose of thyroid, particularly in a man with a count between twenty and forty million per milliliter, should do no harm and may do good.[8]

Androgen has been administered to try to create a "rebound effect." In this therapy the dose is administered for two to three months or longer to depress the sperm count in the hope that it will rebound at an elevated level after the medication is discontinued. This sounds good, in light of similar effects of other hormones on other glands, but the use of androgen works only in some cases and then only for a short while. Some experts report very good results with this treatment,[9] while others caution that there is a danger that it may result in azoospermia, a worse condition than the borderline count which the man had to begin with.[10]

Nonspecific endocrine therapy is currently being tried, but the results are by no means clear. Human chorionic gonadotropin (HCG) has been used in some cases, small doses of cortisone in others. Reports are mixed about the success of these therapies.[11] Finally, clomiphene citrate (Clomid), which is used to treat anovulatory women, has been tried on men. If it can stimulate the pituitary in women to cause ovulation, could it not stimulate the pituitary in men to improve spermatogenesis? Some positive results have been reported, but the results in terms of subsequent pregnancies have not been clear.[12]

Surgery for Certain Problems

There are certain physical problems of the genital organs which may respond to surgery. The most encouraging results for any surgical procedures on the male have been reported in operations for varicocele, varicocelectomies. This condition of dilated testicular veins may be very difficult to diagnose. But once diagnosed, it can be treated surgically with very favorable results, as Dr. Richard Amelar of the New York University Medical School has stressed.[13]

Other conditions which can be operated on are blockages of the tubes in the testicles that carry the sperm out to the penis. These blockages can be congenital, they can be the result of diseases, or they can be caused by vasectomy. The operations for these two conditions have less favorable results than those reported with varicocelectomy. Why are the results less favorable? Doctors are not certain, but they suspect the following reason: when the tubes of the testicles are blocked for whatever reason, sperm are dammed up inside the testicles where they have a tendency to agglutinate or clump together.[14] This tendency may persist even if a path is opened surgically for the sperm to leave the testicle. The sperm that can then be ejaculated still tend to agglutinate, and agglutination is harder to reverse than merely unblocking the path for the sperm.

Husband Artificial Insemination

Husband artificial insemination, or therapeutic insemination with the husband's sperm, is not a treatment for male problems, but it may be chosen in certain highly selected cases in order to get around certain male and female problems. In this procedure the husband's sperm is used to inseminate the wife (as distinct from donor artificial insemination, in which the sperm from an unknown donor is used). In all cases every other possible cause of infertility in the female must be ruled out, with culdoscopy or laparoscopy as the ultimate diagnostic tool. The husband's sperm count must be strong enough so that conception is in the realm of possibility.

The procedure is relatively simple and can be performed in the gynecologist's office, in most cases. The doctor takes a specimen of the husband's sperm and places it in or near the wife's cervix. The procedure must be carefully timed to coincide with the wife's fertile period, based on the monthly Basal Body Temperature Chart and on examination of the cervical mucus. After the sperm has been introduced, the wife remains supine for thirty minutes to an hour to allow maximum penetration. The process is usually repeated twice in one cycle, at forty-eight-hour intervals. It may be tried over a number of different cycles.

When should this procedure be considered? Taymor stresses that it is ". . . best to reserve this therapy as a last resort and also to limit its use to those situations where there is a reasonable chance that it will be of benefit." [15] Many experts feel that these conditions are: the inability of a man to deposit sperm near the woman's cervix; a borderline sperm count; problems with the cervical mucus in the female; and occasionally in cases of extreme retroversion of the uterus, when the uterus is so positioned that the cervix cannot dip into the pool of sperm nearby.

The husband may be unable to deposit sperm near the wife's cervix because of psychological problems such as impotence or premature ejaculation outside the vagina, or because of rarer physical problems such as hypospadias or retrograde ejaculation. Hypospadias is a congenital condition in which the opening of the penis is in such a position that ejaculation occurs downward, and hence sperm is not deposited near the woman's cervix. In this case, artificial insemination may be performed using a specimen of sperm obtained by masturbation. In the rare cases of retrograde ejaculation, in which the sperm collect in the man's bladder rather than being ejaculated out through the penis, the standard treatment to date has been somewhat complicated. The bladder must be emptied and bathed with a special solution to remove all traces of urine before ejaculation. After ejaculation the sperm are collected from the bladder by catheterization, treated, and then placed in the wife's vagina. Sperm are often lost in this procedure, and success rates in terms of subsequent pregnancies have not been high. Recently, however, an alternative therapy has been developed for this condition. Drugs which can stimulate the closing of the neck of the bladder are administered some time before intercourse, and thus the sperm can be ejaculated out through the penis. [16] This would seem to be a more satisfactory treatment, since the sperm do not have to be gathered from the bladder.

Premature ejaculation and impotence respond well to psychotherapy of the behavioral model, and this therapy is the treatment of choice. In certain instances, however, physicians may resort to artificial insemination with the husband's sperm while psychotherapy is going on.

If the male has a borderline sperm count, some doctors might recommend a trial at husband artificial insemination. Two types may be tried, a split ejaculate or a pooled specimen of live and frozen sperm.

The reason for using the split ejaculate is that 75 percent of the motile sperm are found in the first part of an ejaculate. In this procedure, the first part of the husband's specimen is deposited near the wife's cervix, and the rest is deposited in the vagina. Good success rates have been reported by Dr. Richard Amelar using this technique. Before artificial insemination is undertaken, Amelar occasionally advises couples to try this on their own, using a type of coitus interruptus in which the male ejaculates the first part of his sperm near the cervix in the vagina and then withdraws his penis to ejaculate the rest.[17] You should know, however, that not all doctors are in agreement about the efficacy of these techniques.

Pooling of live and frozen sperm has been made possible by very recent improvements in techniques of freezing sperm.[18] Until recently, freezing was possible only with normal sperm counts, but new techniques have obtained better results with borderline counts. These new techniques are most effective in borderline sperm counts where there is good motility.[19] When a pooled specimen is used, the physician usually inseminates the wife with a combination of samples of her husband's sperm — one just obtained by masturbation and one or more previously obtained and then frozen. These new techniques are available only in certain specialized centers. Reported results show that the prognosis is not good: pregnancies have been reported in only 3 to 20 percent of cases.[20]

Finally, husband artificial insemination may be tried if the wife has certain conditions that impede the progress of sperm in her reproductive organs. One of these conditions is an extremely retroverted or tipped uterus. Doctors may first try to reposition the uterus by using a pessary or splint to hold the uterus in a correct position; but if this does not work, artificial insemination may be tried. The other condition that may require artificial insemination is an intractable problem with the mucus of the cervix. After attempting to cure this condition with medication or hormone treatment, the doctor may resort to placing one part of the ejaculate into or beyond the cervical canal so that the sperm may continue on through the uterus into the fallopian tubes. A similar procedure may be followed if the husband has a normal sperm count in the lab but no viable sperm show up in a postcoital test.

Artificial insemination with the husband's sperm does not have a high degree of success except in certain carefully selected cases. If pregnancy does not occur after several trials at husband artificial insemination, the wife should be rechecked for any possible "silent" problems.

PART FIVE

Other Problems

Secondary Infertility

PRIMARY INFERTILITY is not only a complex medical problem but also a wrenching emotional experience. Perhaps even more trying emotionally and equally as complicated medically is another fertility problem: secondary infertility.

Secondary infertility is infertility that occurs after a couple has already had a child. The couple is stunned by the problem because there was no problem before — and there is one child or sometimes more to prove it. Their confident expectations that another baby would arrive have been thwarted. Rather than feeling elated that they have already been able to have one child they feel many of the same emotions that a couple with primary infertility feels. One of my friends went through the same anguish and search for a solution that I did in order to have her third child.

Fifteen percent of all married couples have one child and then find that they are unable to have another one.[1] Yet their glands and reproductive organs functioned perfectly adequately before. What happens to cause infertility after they have proved their capacity for fertility?

It is easier for physicians to determine what is *not* causing their infertility, because the previous pregnancy has demonstrated the capacity of certain organs to perform. Hence, congenital malformations of the reproductive organs can usually be ruled out.

Similarly, severe chromosomal abnormalities can also usually be ruled out. What then can cause secondary infertility?

Aging may be a simple, but cruel, explanation; certain women simply undergo early menopause, sometimes as early as age thirty-five.[2] Other conditions can develop — diseases, severe dietary deficiencies, injuries, and a host of other problems that the human animal is heir to. Secondary infertility is just as complicated as primary infertility, and for this reason, a couple with secondary infertility must have the same thorough workups as those described in Chapters 7–10.

The male may develop three principal problems: those involving the transport of sperm from the testicle out to the penis; problems in the production of sperm; and psychological problems that prevent him from having intercourse.

Physical problems with the transport of sperm are usually related to blockages of the vas deferens. These obstructions can be caused by genital tuberculosis and by gonorrhea, so any onset of these diseases since the last pregnancy must be suspect. Injury to the testicles can also be responsible for problems of secondary infertility.

Problems with the production of sperm can arise for any number of reasons mentioned in Chapter 9. Diseases which have occurred since the last pregnancy, like mumps orchitis, or viral illness with a high fever, may impair spermatogenesis. Environmental factors such as excess exposure of the testicles to heat or radiation may play a role. Extreme fatigue or extreme stress can drastically lower the sperm count, as can be demonstrated in the case of a man whose sperm count dropped to nil for eight months following a severe automobile accident in which two other passengers were killed.[3] Finally, medication for other problems may adversely affect spermatogenesis, as mentioned in Chapter Nine. These drugs are anticancer and antimicrobial drugs and certain steroids.

Psychological problems that cause impotence, premature ejaculation, or ejaculatory incompetence may arise after an earlier pregnancy, but they are so far-ranging in number and in possible cause that it would be impossible to enumerate them here. Men should be forewarned, however, that occasionally these conditions may be attributed to psychological problems when they are actually a result of drugs and medications or of certain diseases, such as diabetes and hypothyroidism. Impotence is frequent in narcotics addicts. Excessive use of various types of tranquilizers and certain antihypertensive drugs can also cause impotence.

The female may also develop problems, some of which may be directly related to an earlier pregnancy. Those most likely to be linked to an earlier pregnancy are damage or infection of the cervix and blockages of the fallopian tubes caused by a minor infection after pregnancy. If the first pregnancy has been an ectopic pregacy, one that implants outside the uterus in a fallopian tube or even in the abdominal cavity, physicians might suspect a possible problem with the tubes. If the ectopic pregnancy has ruptured, it may have caused damage to the ovaries or the fallopian tubes, and this damage may make it more difficult for a woman to conceive again.

Other problems which may arise are: infections of the vagina or cervix; cervical polyps, which block the opening of the cervix; fibroid tumors of the uterus; or blocked fallopian tubes, which are either a result of infection following the earlier pregnancy or a result of diseases like gonorrhea or tuberculosis. A woman may also develop psychological problems that interfere with the complex endocrinological mechanisms involved in ovulation. And she *could* develop endometriosis, although this disease is most often found in women who have never borne children. All of these problems have treatments, as described in Chapter 12. But the patient is urged to seek out the same thorough evaluation and the same expert treatment she would if she had primary infertility.

CHAPTER 16

Habitual Miscarriage

No SINGLE problem within the field of infertility is as much argued as habitual miscarriage, or habitual abortion, as it is known medically. Some authorities resist defining habitual miscarriage as a specific medical problem. They tend to see successive miscarriages as the random but unfortunately coincidental turning of the wheel of fortune. After all, they argue, miscarriage occurs in 10 percent of all pregnancies. Even the authorities who agree that there is, in fact, such a medical problem are not agreed on its causes or its treatments. Hence, I will present here the few ideas that are generally accepted about habitual miscarriage and some of the hypotheses that abound about both cause and treatment.

Habitual miscarriers are women who conceive easily but are unable to carry pregnancy to term at least three times in succession. I can only try to imagine their sorrow. *I* grieved for myself, for my husband, and for our failure. But the woman who habitually miscarries grieves for more than herself and her husband. A life was there within her, waiting to be born. Her grief, each time, is for the loss of a living being — as well as for her inability to nurture that life successfully.

The outlook for these women is not hopeless. In a recent review of the subject, Drs. Carl Tupper and Robert Weil have concluded that subsequent successful pregnancy may occur in as many as 80 percent of these women with varying treatments.[1]

Some Recognized Causes of
Habitual Miscarriage

Given the general disagreement among specialists, what are the most commonly accepted causes of habitual miscarriage? They fall into two categories: first, the same causes which are responsible for the isolated miscarriages that occur in 10 percent of all pregnancies; and second, definable physical problems with the female reproductive organs.

What, then, are the causes of isolated miscarriage? The two most generally cited ones are: the faulty development of the embryo and the incorrect implantation of the embryo in the lining of the uterus, the endometrium. In the first instance, the embryo may fail to develop properly because there is some chromosomal abnormality in the sperm or the egg. Since it cannot develop properly into a normal human being, it aborts spontaneously; and physicians often offer some comfort by rightly stressing that this is nature's way of taking care of the health of the species. In the second instance, the fertilized egg may not implant properly in the lining of the uterus. It thus does not make the proper connection with the mother's life system, it cannot be properly nourished, and it aborts spontaneously. Treatment for the first problem has not yet been developed, and may never be, but there are a variety of theories about treatment of the second problem which will be discussed below.

What are the physical problems with the reproductive organs that cause habitual miscarriage? Most doctors agree on three principal problems. The first is congenital malformation of the uterus, a condition that occurs only in a small percentage of women. Rather than having a normal pear-shaped uterus which can expand as the baby grows, these women have uteruses of different shapes that cannot enlarge enough to accommodate a growing baby. The second problem is a weak or incompetent cervix, again a relatively rare condition in which the cervix is not strong enough to remain closed tightly as the weight of the uterus above it becomes greater. The cervix therefore dilates too easily, and the baby is miscarried. The third problem which can cause habitual miscarriage is the presence of uterine growths. Severe fibroid tumors of the uterus, which are benign fibrous growths, apparently can prevent the implantation of a fertilized egg. Endometrial polyps, small growths of tissue on the lining of the uterus, can also prevent implantation.

All of these are clearly diagnosable physical problems, although the first two may not be diagnosed until after miscarriage has occurred, and hysterosalpingography may be necessary to diagnose congenital malformations of the uterus. Surgery may be recommended for these problems. Some congenital malformations of the uterus can be corrected by reconstructive surgery. A weak cervix can be strengthened by use of tight encircling sutures or a silastic ring which are removed just prior to labor and delivery. Endometrial polyps and fibroid tumors can be excised surgically in many instances, but surgery should be as conservative as possible in order to preserve as much of the childbearing function of the uterus as possible. Unfortunately hysterectomy is all too readily advised for fibroid tumors. You should know that more conservative surgery is available for certain cases of fibroid tumors, the myomectomy described on page 98.

It is advisable that these surgical procedures be performed before another pregnancy has begun. In some rare cases, a woman who is threatening to miscarry because of incompetent cervix may be helped to carry that pregnancy to term by an operation to encircle the cervix with sutures or with a silastic ring.[2]

Controversial Causes

Extremely Retroverted Uterus.

There is a great deal of disagreement about whether this condition is in fact causative in habital miscarriage. Kleegman and Kaufman feel that it can be, in some cases,[3] but others do not always agree. In this condition the uterus is so drastically flexed forward or backward that it does not have the proper space to expand in as the baby grows. Some doctors recommend placing a pessary or splint inside the vagina to support the uterus in the correct position. If this fails, surgery to correct the position of the uterus, a uterine suspension, can be undertaken.

There are five other causes of habitual miscarriage about which there is even less general agreement.[4]

Defective Germ Cells

Researchers have queried whether couples who have the problem of habitual miscarriage might not have a higher than average incidence of defective sperm or eggs. Some research seems to confirm this, at least in the case of men, as sperm are easier to study than the eggs are. This research has shown a slightly higher number of abnormally shaped sperm in the sperm analyses of men whose wives are habitual miscarriers. Authorities hypothesize that there might be a similarly high incidence of defective eggs in the woman who is a habitual miscarrier, but to date, less research has been carried out on this subject.

Hormonal Deficiencies

Deficiencies in thyroid, estrogen, and progesterone have all been cited as the possible causes of habitual miscarriage. Thyroid deficiency can be clearly measured and treated with thyroid medication. Estrogen deficiency is more difficult to assess, but some doctors recommend treatment with synthetic estrogen *prior* to pregnancy to "prime the endometrium."[5] Luteal-phase deficiencies, or progesterone deficiencies, have long been accepted as a common cause of habitual miscarriage. The woman fails to produce enough progesterone to stimulate the growth of an adequate lining of the uterus. In these cases, the fertilized egg passes out of the uterus quite early, and the lost pregnancy may be detectable only by careful examination of the Basal Body Temperature Charts or laboratory studies. Treatment with dosages of progesterone and careful assessment of progesterone levels have been recommended and used to maintain pregnancies. But in recent years, doctors have begun to question the statistics on this treatment, and some have even suggested that the prognosis may be just as good without progesterone.[6] Doctors may be growing more conservative about advising the use of hormonal preparations to avert miscarriages because of recent reports about the long-term effects of similar drugs. One such drug, diethylstilbestrol (DES), was used in the fifties in women who were threatening to miscarry. The miscarriages were prevented, but some of the children of these women have developed health problems.

Immunologic Incompatibility

It has long been recognized that an Rh negative mother can develop antibodies to the Rh positive factor after she has had one Rh positive child. These antibodies can cause problems in subsequent pregnancies with Rh positive fetuses, either causing stillbirth late in pregnancy or a disease of the blood in the newborn infant. A treatment now exists for this problem, in which the mother receives medication immediately following the birth of her first Rh positive child so that she will not develop antibodies which would cause an immune reaction and stillbirth in subsequent pregnancies. This well-defined immunologic problem has been conquered, but its existence has suggested that habitual miscarriers may have some other, as yet undiscovered, immunologic incompatibilities which cause them to miscarry their fetuses. Drs. Tupper and Weil feel that this is one of the most important areas where research is being carried out.[7]

Psychological Problems

Clearly all psychological problems do not cause habitual miscarriage. Otherwise, habitual miscarriage would be far more common than it is. However, some authorities suggest that, in certain women, psychological upsets work through the hypothalamic-pituitary network to affect adversely the hormonal balance necessary to sustain a pregnancy. Moreover, with all the data emerging about chemical imbalances in certain psychological problems, one would wonder if some chemical factor associated with a psychological upset could not also be at work causing habitual miscarriage.

Dietary Deficiencies

Some researchers have suggested that dietary or vitamin deficiencies can cause habitual miscarriage, but this is the most controversial theory of all. It is true that diet is extremely important for the pregnant woman. However, after reviewing the literature on the subject, Drs. Tupper and Weil have found no conclusive proof that dietary deficiencies are involved in the problem of habitual miscarriage.[8]

Clearly, doctors have just begun to define and solve the problem of habitual miscarriage. Solutions are available only for the physical problems of the reproductive organs and for problems with the Rh factor. The other problems await clarification.

If all this seems unduly vague to the woman who is a habitual miscarrier, a few general words of advice can be offered. Seek a doctor who does feel that habitual miscarriage is a specific problem requiring intense investigation and specific treatment. Seek other opinions from specialists in infertility if a hysterectomy is recommended for any reason. Undergo a thorough examination and persist in your treatment. Expect that, whatever treatment is prescribed for you, you will also probably have to conform to the old-time standard treatment for miscarriage as well: abstinence from intercourse, bed rest, and avoidance of all extreme physical exertion.

CHAPTER 17

Irresolvable Infertility: Options and Alternatives

AFTER a thorough and complete infertility workup, you may have been able to find the cause of your problem and to obtain some treatment. If you are lucky enough to have conceived, you feel a boundless gratitude to those who helped you. But one of you may have found a cause that to date has no real solution. Or you may be among those in whom no apparent cause can be found. You are understandably disheartened, but at least you know you have had the fullest examinations possible. And your knowledge makes you better able to decide what alternative you will choose now: adoption, artificial insemination with a donor's sperm, or continuing to build a life without children. If you decide on either of the first two alternatives, you should set a definite date when you will initiate adoption procedures or insemination treatments.

Adoption

You should obtain information about adoption from your physician or from a number of different agencies, both local and national.[1] Such agencies can best inform you about the availability of adoptable children in your area.

It is true that fewer children are available for adoption, partially because of the increase in effective contraceptive measures, partially because of the number of legal abortions, and partially because some unwed mothers are choosing to keep their children. You may have to wait a long time. You may decide to adopt abroad. You may decide to adopt an older child or a child with problems. But the possibility of adoption is real in most areas.

"If we adopt, will we then have a child of our own?" We have all heard of pregnancies following adoption. The parents to whom this happens can consider themselves doubly blessed. The idea is so widespread that several eminent infertility experts have conducted research to determine if, in fact, adoption does increase a couple's chances of conceiving.[2] These studies have suggested that it does not. However, as Dr. John Rock and his colleagues have stated,[3] adoption certainly does not appear to prevent a woman from becoming pregnant.

Artificial Insemination with a Donor's Sperm

Another option is available for a highly selected group of infertile couples. If all possible causes of infertility have been ruled out in the female and a male factor has been found, the couple may want to consider artificial insemination with a donor's sperm. This is an extremely delicate matter. Both partners must be enthusiastic about it. Absolute honesty is essential here, as any hesitancy whatsoever is sufficient reason not to select the treatment. The husband should not agree only because he thinks it will make his wife happy.

The technique is the same as that used for artificial insemination with the husband's sperm, but in this instance the sperm is obtained from a donor known only to the physician. The donor is carefully selected in order to try to eliminate the possibility of congenital or genetic problems. In some cases the donor is chosen because he has coloring and build like the husband's. Some doctors habitually mix some of the husband's sperm with the donor's; others advise the couple to have intercourse the night of the procedure.

The prime advantage of this technique is that the wife is able to bear a child. It is natural, however, that many couples should have reservations about this. If either spouse has any reservations, the method should not be considered.

Even in carefully selected cases the success rate is only 50 to 60 percent. If no pregnancy occurs after several months of inseminations, the woman should once more be examined to determine if she has any possible cause of infertility, as yet undiscovered.

Donor artificial insemination has been received with mixed reactions. When it was first performed in the early twentieth century, there was an outcry in medical circles. In the last thirty years, the procedure has become more widespread. However, its status is far from clear. The Roman Catholic church rejects it, and the Orthodox Jewish faith opposes it. It also has a very cloudy legal status. Some doctors advise the completion of numerous legal documents by the wife and husband before the procedure is performed. Others advise immediate adoption of the child by the husband. Still other doctors perform the insemination and then send a woman to an obstetrician who knows nothing about the procedure and so assumes that the husband has fathered the child. Other doctors feel that secrecy is so important that no documents are signed. To date, a few suits have been brought before the courts. A recent case in California involved a husband who refused child support for a child born as the result of donor artificial insemination, even though he had signed a paper giving his consent at the time. The lower courts declared he was not responsible for the child's support, but the state supreme court reversed the lower court's decision.[4] In this case, and in a few others, the courts have decided that the husband who agrees to his wife's artificial insemination by a donor is to be considered the father of the child. However, there is no law to this effect on the books.

Choosing Childlessness

You may decide to continue to build your life without children. Indeed, in today's world, where many couples are voluntarily choosing not to have children, there is no longer the same stigma attached to the childless state that there once was.

If you make this decision, do so positively. Plan to fill your life to the brim. If you find you are depressed about your childless state, seek help from a friend, a member of the clergy, or a psychiatrist. If you find that you want contact with children or young people, there are many ways you can manage this through family or friends, through work, or by participating in any number of youth organizations.

The women's liberation movement has helped women to realize that their sole function in life is not to bear children, that child-rearing years are limited within the total life span, that there are countless creative ways to find fulfillment. Indeed, there *are* options and alternatives to having children.

PART SIX

The Future
of Infertility

What is the future of infertility? We all wish that it, like cancer, would disappear, conquered by medical science. But the world's problem of overpopulation and the infertile couple's problem of underpopulation will not be easily solved.

Two issues seem particularly pressing. Are there ways infertility can be prevented? Certain problems are clearly out of our control, like congenital anomalies and chromosomal abnormalities, to name only two. Nonetheless, women, in particular, must be educated to weigh the risks of various contraceptive measures and to choose that measure which is least risky for them. Women must learn the chance they are taking in deferring childbirth. They must know the problems associated with certain diseases. They must learn the advantages of conservative pelvic surgery. And they must learn to express their opinions clearly and unequivocally to their doctors.

The second issue is less personal and more global. With the problem of overpopulation growing each year, some doctors are beginning to advocate an end to research on infertility. They argue that the funds supporting infertility research should be diverted to support research on ever more efficacious contraceptive measures. They argue that the dangers to the world caused by overpopulation are far more significant than the mere joy brought to the few infertile couples who are enabled to bear children. And moreover, they argue, infertility is not life-threatening. To these researchers, we who have suffered with infertility can only respond humbly, pleading: Continue the research.

CHAPTER 18

Birth Control Measures and Infertility

ONE of the major advances in the twentieth century has been the development of reliable methods of birth control. These contraceptive measures have freed women of the burden of unwanted children, have made possible the planning and spacing of children, and have contributed to the solution of the staggering problem of overpopulation.

At the same time, however, effective contraceptive measures have raised other questions. Women no longer run the risk of disease and damage to their bodies caused by multiple pregnancies; but now they are beginning to wonder about — and to discover — the diseases and damage to their bodies that can be caused by certain contraceptives. Women no longer need to fear that their education or professional training will be ended because of a surprise pregnancy; but now they are starting to learn that, for some, deferring childbearing too long may mean deferring it forever.

No medication can enter our body, no medical intervention can be made without the risk of some adverse side effects. Birth control measures are no exception, as so many recent reports have pointed out. Increased risk of heart attacks and thrombophlebitis are the most widely publicized adverse effects of the oral contraceptives, but there are others. And the other methods of birth control also have their measure of adverse effects.

Most important for us, we must examine the question of the relationship between birth control measures and infertility. Can the contraceptives we use to plan our families affect our future ability to have children? The evidence is by no means clear. There is much debate among doctors. Many argue that the benefits to thousands of women of easy and effective contraception far outweigh the disadvantage of infertility which may be caused in only a few women. Here are the views of some authorities on the relationships of certain contraceptive measures to the future fertility of the user.

Chemical Contraceptives:
The Pill and The Injectable

Oral contraceptives are hormone preparations which prevent conception by interfering with ovulation. Doctors have long been aware that certain women discover infertility problems on discontinuing the pill. In 20 percent of these women, ovulation does not return for as long as three months after discontinuing the pill.[1] In 2 to 5 percent of these women, ovulation does not return for as long as a year.[2] C. R. Garcia and other authorities feel that this state of anovulation after using the birth control pill is not caused by the pill but is probably evidence that the woman's anovulation existed before she began using the pill.[3]

In almost all cases, it is possible to restimulate ovulation using the hormonal preparations described on pages 106–109. It should be recalled, however, that even these preparations — Clomid and Pergonal — carry with them certain risks. I therefore agree with Dr. W. C. Andrews, who states: "It would appear prudent to avoid protracted ovulation suppression in patients who have evidenced gross ovarian deficiency and who do not have at least a modest family." [4]

The most recent experiments in the field of oral contraception have been with chemical contraceptives that contain ingredients similar to those in the pills, but which are given by injection and intended to last over a long period of time, from one to three months. These are only in the experimental stages, and little has been reported about long-term side effects. Currently they are not on the market as a contraceptive, and this seems wise. Given the continuing revelation of adverse side effects of the oral contraceptives, I wonder if the future may not reveal a similar group of adverse side effects for the injectable, long-lasting contraceptives.

The Intrauterine Contraceptive Devices: The IUD

The IUDs are devices inserted into the uterus which prevent conception in a high percentage of cases. No one is sure just exactly how the IUDs work, but they may interfere with the implantation of the fertilized egg. There are many kinds of intrauterine devices: rings, coils, shields, loops, to name only a few. And they are made from a variety of materials, including polyurethane and copper.

Dr. Hugh Davis of Johns Hopkins University, an authority on the IUD, has maintained that fertility rates after the use of the IUD have been "comparable to those observed after the discontinuation of other birth control methods . . ." [5] However, other doctors have reported and documented other adverse side effects of the IUDs which certainly could affect fertility.

Some doctors have documented an increased incidence of pelvic inflammatory disease (PID) in users of IUDs.[6] In its severe stages, pelvic inflammatory disease can cause infection or inflammation of the fallopian tubes, and this damage to the fallopian tubes can cause infertility, as described on pages 102–103. Davis, who is an advocate of the IUD, is skeptical of the reports of increased incidence of pelvic inflammatory disease in the users of the IUDs. He argues that the PID could be a result of other factors and not directly related to the IUD. He maintains that: *"Unless a documented febrile illness follows immediately on the heels of the insertion procedure, a cause-and-effect relationship with the IUD is unlikely.* [Davis' italics]" [7] It should also be noted that the device most frequently associated with the reported acute cases of PID, the Dalkon Shield, has been removed from the market.[8] Nonetheless, women should see a physician immediately if they develop a high fever after the insertion of any IUD.

The second adverse side effect of the IUD is an increased incidence of ectopic pregnancy, but this occurs only rarely.[9] When the device fails and pregnancy occurs, women using the IUD are six times more likely to have ectopic pregnancies than women using other contraceptives.[10] The IUD does not actually cause the ectopic pregnancy, but because the device is inserted in the uterus, it cannot prevent the implantation of a fertilized egg outside the uterus. As described on page 131, ectopic pregnancy can cause damage to the fallopian tubes or ovaries, which can result in subsequent problems with fertility. Technically, the IUD would not be responsible for the fertility problem, but the ectopic pregnancy would.

Tubal Ligation and Vasectomy

Tubal ligation and vasectomy are usually undertaken when a woman or man has already had children and wants a permanent effective contraceptive. In tubal ligation, a woman's fallopian tubes are tied, bound surgically so that the sperm cannot pass through them. In vasectomy, the vas deferens in each testicle is cut so that sperm cannot pass through them.

If, for whatever reason, people who have had these operations decide they want to undo them, they find themselves faced with infertility. The only course in either case is surgery, in which the affected part of the tubes is excised and the clean ends are sewn together. Results in the female are not encouraging. Reported results in the male have been more encouraging, for newly developed microsurgery techniques seem to have improved the prognosis.[11] But men who have had vasectomy may have developed agglutination of their sperm,[12] as described on page 123. And agglutination is a problem that, to date, has no solution.

Because the reported results are somewhat discouraging, both men and women are advised to undergo vasectomy or tubal ligation only when they are *absolutely* certain they want no more children.

Physical Barriers to Conception:
The Diaphragm and The Condom

The oldest form of mechanical contraception is a physical barrier which prevents sperm and egg from meeting. The condom has been documented since 1564 when the great Italian anatomist and authority on syphilis, Gabriel Fallopius, claimed to have invented a sheath of linen to cover the penis during intercourse.[13] Since that time, linen has given way to rubber and plastic, and the condom continues to be widely used throughout the world.[14] A similar barrier device for females, the diaphragm, was invented in the late nineteenth century, and until the discovery of oral contraception, it was widely used. According to some experts, the diaphragm seems to be making a comeback today.

The condom covers the penis during intercourse and catches the sperm which are ejaculated. The diaphragm, lubricated with spermicidal jelly, is inserted into the vagina to cover the cervix and prevent sperm from entering the cervix. The condom, when properly used, is effective, and with newly developed materials, there is little danger that it will break. The diaphragm, when properly fitted and properly used, is 95 percent effective. And no major adverse side effects have been reported with either device.

Unequivocally, it can be stated that the condom and the diaphragm cannot be connected with infertility. They do not cause anovulation. They are not associated with increased incidence of PID or of ectopic pregnancy. And both of them have other advantages. The condom can actually prevent or dramatically lessen the transmission of venereal disease. The diaphragm can protect the cervix from infection and injury during coitus.[15]

But both condom and diaphragm require forethought. They

are a nuisance to many people. They can be messy. They can interrupt the spontaneity of love-making. They are not absolutely 100 percent effective.

In my opinion, however, the physical-barrier contraceptive methods have definite advantages. They pose no risk whatsoever to future fertility. They do have positive side effects. Even doctors agree that they are the least risky of all contraceptive measures in terms of future adverse side effects.

CHAPTER 19

Can Infertility Be Prevented?

Is it possible to prevent infertility — or, at least, to minimize one's chances of encountering it? The answer is yes and no. Clearly, at present, there is no way to prevent a congenital anomaly of the uterus or the congenital absence of sperm. But there are ways to avoid gonorrhea, for example. And one can choose a low-risk method of birth control. Education about other aspects of fertility and infertility can enable us all to choose paths with the fewest risks for future fertility.

Health in Childhood

Preventing infertility begins in childhood, for boys as well as for girls. In boys, the scrotum should be carefully examined routinely to uncover cases of undescended testes. These must be operated on, brought down out of the body into the scrotum when the boy is between the ages of five and eight. Otherwise, prolonged exposure to the body's heat will permanently impair spermatogenesis. A second cause of sterility in men, post-pubertal mumps orchitis, can now be avoided. Mumps vaccine should be routinely given to any male who passes into puberty without ever having had mumps in childhood.

In childhood and throughout their lives, girls should be thoroughly and routinely examined for problems that might lead to future infertility, particularly in cases of suspected appendicitis. A ruptured appendix and ensuing peritonitis can cause damage to the fallopian tubes. In adolescent girls and women, the diagnosis of acute appendicitis is often difficult to make, because the symptom of pelvic pain can be caused by any number of problems, including pain at the time of ovulation.

The sexual development of girls should also be carefully watched. The delayed onset of menstruation, especially past the age of sixteen, should be thoroughly investigated. Extremely irregular menstrual periods should also be carefully checked.

Finally, any woman who has had ovulatory and menstrual irregularities should be advised not to use the oral contraceptives as a method of birth control. The use of the pill would simply mask already existing problems, as discussed on page 35.

Sex Education

The importance of sex education cannot be overestimated, not only for the psychosexual well-being of people but also for their future fertility.

Early education about venereal diseases is imperative, as gonorrhea can cause infertility in both sexes, damaging the fallopian tubes in women and the testicular tubules that transport sperm in men. This disease is particularly a problem because of its rapid increase in recent years. Since the disease is curable, many young people simply do not worry about it. They reason that they will be able to get treatment if they happen to get gonorrhea. But what if they have a strain of gonococcus resistant to penicillin? What if they miss the symptoms? Girls should be warned that females can have gonorrhea that presents no symptoms whatsoever until it is in a very advanced stage. The positive advantages of condoms as a means of protecting against the transmission of venereal disease should be emphasized. And the dangers of sterility following severe cases of gonorrhea should be stressed.

Early education about pregnancy is also important, first and obviously so that young people can learn how to avoid unwanted pregnancy but also so that they can learn how pregnancy and abortion can affect future fertility. Most young people are fully aware that they want to avoid pregnancy, but they may not be adequately educated about contraceptive methods. They may find themselves pregnant and facing an abortion. The dangers of back-street abortions must be stressed in sex education classes. An illegal or aseptic abortion, complicated by infection, may endanger the life of the woman and threaten her future fertility. The illegal abortion must be avoided at all costs. Sex educators should stress, nonetheless, that mild infections occurring even after a septic abortion should be treated immediately to avoid damage to the fallopian tubes and subsequent fertility problems. It is, of course, far better to avoid pregnancy altogether.

Birth control measures should also be carefully explained to teenagers. Young people should learn how these can be used to avoid the risk of pregnancy. But they should also be fully apprised of the hazards and benefits of the different types of contraceptive measures.

Delayed Childbearing

More and more women are choosing to have fewer children and to begin their families later in life, after education is over and career begun. In the 1970s this choice is safer than it has been in the past, for defects like Down's syndrome, which are more likely to occur in the fetuses of older women, can be diagnosed by amniocentesis, a procedure in which amniotic fluid is removed from the uterus and examined to determine if there are any detectable defects in the fetus. But amniocentesis does not solve all the problems.

Women should be aware that they are making a series of wagers in deferring childbearing. They are betting first of all against time. Their fertility declines each year, but especially after the age of 35. Menopause can begin in some women at age 35, in even more women at 40. And to date, there are no ways to predict just which women will have this early menopause.

They are also betting against disease. Obviously, the longer you live, the more opportunity you have of contracting any number of diseases. Where fertility is concerned, the dangers of diseases like gonorrhea and tuberculosis have already been stressed. But there are other problems which threaten fertility and which are more likely to occur the older you are. Fibroid tumors are more common and less easy to excise surgically in women over thirty. And endometriosis which can wreak such havoc on the pelvic organs is more likely to occur in women in their late twenties who have put off having children.

When faced with the onset of these diseases, women naturally want to feel "It won't cause infertility in *me.*" But the experience of one local gynecologist is worth recording. In his years of practice, he has routinely advised women with endometriosis to try to begin their families immediately. He often hears that a career is in progress, that the time is not quite right, and so forth. But in a high percentage of cases, he sees the same women two to three years later as patients with infertility. They have decided that the time is right, but nature has decided otherwise.

In addition, women who defer childbearing are betting against the risks of treatment, for certain procedures to cure gynecological problems carry some risks. Those used for infections of the cervix, a common malady, are one example. Physicians often treat these cervical infections with electrocauterization or occasionally with a minor surgical procedure known as conization to cut away the infected part of the cervix. These two procedures can cure the cervical infection but may permanently impair the ability of the cervix to produce an adequate supply of that mucus which is necessary and favorable to sperm at the time of ovulation.

The treatment of other pelvic disorders can also threaten future fertility. If a patient has to undergo pelvic surgery for any reason, she should firmly insist that the surgery be as conservative as possible, and she should seek a second opinion if hysterectomy is advised as discussed on page 106. Some doctors advise hysterectomy for fibroid tumors; you should know that myomectomy is possible in certain cases. Some doctors advise hysterectomy for endometriosis; you should know that other procedures to treat the problem are available. Some doctors advise removing the fallopian tube or ovary where an ectopic pregnancy has implanted; you should know that in some cases, with conservative surgery, it is possible to salvage the tube or the ovary.

Male Problems

There seems to be less that a male can do to insure his fertility and to avoid infertility. But he should avoid the enemies of spermatogenesis whenever possible: disease, certain drugs, and a few environmental problems.

Both men and women should avoid gonorrhea altogether, but if the disease is contracted or even exposure suspected, immediate treatment should be sought. Tuberculosis should also be treated speedily. If a man has gone through puberty without ever having had mumps, he should obtain mumps vaccine. He should know which medications can adversely affect spermatogenesis (see pages 73–74). He should know that his fertility might be affected by individual intolerances to tobacco, alcohol, and drugs. And he should definitely avoid exposure of the testicles to x ray, to excessive heat, or to injury.

CHAPTER 20

More Will Be Done

A FEW decades ago, only 10 percent of infertile couples could be helped. Many of the diagnostic tests and treatments described in the preceding chapters had not even been developed. Nineteen forty-four saw the invention of culdoscopy by Decker, 1946 saw the development of the fern test by Papanicolaou. The late 1950s saw the fundamental research on ovulation-inducing drugs. In recent years, there has been work on improved surgical techniques, finer hormonal tests, and more. Today 40 to 50 percent of all infertile couples can be helped to bear children. Tomorrow even more may be helped. Current research is being pursued in many different areas, some of it controversial, some of it well accepted.

Male Problems

Research continues on methods of stimulating spermatogenesis and improving sperm counts, but a solution seems very far away.

Greater promise is given in two other areas: microsurgery and improved techniques of freezing sperm. Improvement in microsurgery provides greater accuracy in surgery for blockages of the tubes that transport sperm in the testicles.[1] And improved techniques of freezing sperm may make possible the preservation of motility which, to date, has been such a problem in borderline sperm counts.[2] This, in turn, would open the door to a greater possibility of pregnancy following the insemination of a woman with a pool of a number of frozen specimens of her husband's sperm.

Female Problems

The problem of faulty ovulation has been solved for some women by Clomid and Pergonal. For others, however, new research on the relationship between the hypothalamus and the pituitary may promise new hope.[3]

The greatest dilemmas that remain in the infertile female are physical problems of the reproductive organs, particularly irresolvable blockages of the fallopian tubes. To solve these researchers have been investigating both the use of artificial organs and the transplant of living organs.

Japanese and Australian physicians have experimented with artificial fallopian tubes made of polyurethane.[4] However, no pregnancies have been reported. The artificial oviduct may fail because it cannot be made to imitate the wavelike motions of the cilia in the human fallopian tube, nor can it contain the same secretions.

Transplantation of the fallopian tubes has been undertaken most recently in South Africa. But again, there have been no reports of subsequent pregnancies. In addition to the risk of rejection of a transplanted organ,[5] there are also problems with guaranteeing full physiologic functioning of the tubes.

Transplants of the uterus and ovaries have also been discussed as possible ways to cure certain infertile women. But to date, experiments have been performed only on animals.[6] A strong argument has been made against transplantations of ovaries in particular, because this, in essence, would involve transplanting someone else's genetic history into a different woman.[7] The ethical considerations are great, and the notion of 1984 rings too strongly with some people.

One other area of research offers great promise. This is the laboratory culture of human germ cells, research being carried out by Drs. Edwards, Purdy, and Steptoe at Cambridge University in England.[8] Their research might solve the problem of irresolvable blockage of the fallopian tubes or even of unexplained infertility. An egg removed from the woman at just the right moment would be fertilized with her husband's sperm in a test tube and then implanted in the same woman's uterus. Edwards, Purdy, and Steptoe's recent report is cautiously optimistic that some day their research will help couples who today cannot be helped.

For infertile couples, it is a blessing that research on infertility continues in the face of the population explosion. While one cannot underestimate the dangers of overpopulation, physicians must continue to consider the miseries of childless couples. We *should* aim toward a world in which each adult merely replaces him- or herself, but it is humane to hope that *all* those who suffer from infertility may one day have this opportunity.

A Child Is Born

MY HUSBAND and I were fortunate — fortunate that we finally found a doctor who could make the diagnosis, fortunate that my condition could be treated, fortunate that our surgeon was an expert. But the greatest fortune of all was that, given a 60 to 70 percent chance of failure, we were lucky enough to succeed.

Pregnancy came as a surprise. We had resigned ourselves to a life without children. And even when my period was three weeks late, I was not convinced. When the lab report finally came back positive, my husband and I were both overjoyed.

But after the initial elation, I began to feel like a fragile container with a precious breakable object inside. I was afraid to move, afraid some misstep would jar the baby out of me. When I saw my doctor, my anxieties were confirmed.

I heard the door open as he walked into the room, and I burst out, "Congratulations, Doctor. You did it! I'm pregnant."

"No, Mrs. Harrison," he said. "You and your husband did it! Congratulations to you!"

After examining me and muttering a terse "Excellent," his initial jubilance changed. He wrote a prescription for vitamins, and then growled ominously, "No hard physical exertion. Don't move furniture. And no sex for three months!"

After all those months of seemingly endless intercourse to get pregnant, now it had to stop altogether. Could intercourse cause me to miscarry?

The first three months were agonizing. We knew that if a miscarriage were to occur, it would most likely come in that first trimester. We kept the secret of my pregnancy to ourselves, not even telling our families. We were afraid that just letting out the news might jinx us in some way.

I worried over everything I did. Was this package too heavy? Could I risk any mild form of sexual involvement? Was I eating the right foods? Would a cold affect the baby? And, when I got a strep throat, I imagined all sorts of dire repercussions. I guess all pregnant women feel this way, but I had no assurance that I could *ever* get pregnant again.

The first three months passed. And I breathed a sigh of relief: out of the first danger zone. And sex could resume. But even then, I could not really throw myself into it. I kept wondering what the thrusting would do. Could I have an orgasm? What if . . . ?

I also went through a phase of wondering if the baby was really there. Was my pregnancy just imaginary? My stomach stayed flat as a pancake, as much as I wanted it to balloon out. But then one day, late in July, I felt a flutter. And from then on, there was a third member of our family.

Summer passed into fall, fall into the beginning of winter. Natural childbirth classes began, along with sessions with a doctor specialized in the hypnotic control of pain. In order to help me relax, he told me to imagine the most beautiful scene possible. And all I could think of was a wriggling, healthy baby being held up by one foot uttering its first wail.

Six weeks later my imaginary scene became a reality — a boy. And . . . he had fingers, and toes. Eyes, and ears. Lungs, and legs, and arms. We simply could not believe it.

All our years of searching, all the frustrations of misdiagnosis, all the anger between us, all the pain of surgery — all this had ended in success. We have one child, who seems to us a miracle, arriving as he did just a few days before Christmas. It now looks as if we may never be able to have another child. But we are overjoyed. For one brief moment, two years ago, one sperm and one egg finally met and joined. We are humbled that we should have been so lucky.

Out of our search, out of our pain, and out of our joy has come this book — with the hope that it may help all of you to find the treatment you deserve and that it may help some of you to have the child you want.

Appendices
Illustrations
Notes
Selected Bibliography
Glossary of Medical
  Terms
Index

Evaluation of the Woman

Basic Preliminary Workup

1. Detailed medical history and physical examination (pp. 55–56).
2. Menstrual and sexual history (pp. 56–58).
3. Pelvic examination (p. 58): visual examination of the external genitalia, vagina, and cervix and manual examination of the cervix, uterus, and ovaries.
4. Laboratory studies of blood, urine, and thyroid function (p. 59).
5. Basal Body Temperature Charts (pp. 59–60 and Fig. 5): chart of a woman's body temperature, taken on arising and recorded daily throughout the menstrual cycle. One of the tests to determine the presence or absence of ovulation.
6. Endometrial biopsy (pp. 60–61): minor surgical procedure in which a piece of the lining of the uterus (the endometrium) is removed, treated chemically, and examined under a microscope. One of the tests to determine the presence or absence of ovulation and the production of progesterone.
7. Tubal insufflation or Rubin test (pp. 64–66): a test to determine if the fallopian tubes are open. Carbon dioxide is passed into the uterus and its pressure is checked to determine if it passes out of the uterus through the fallopian tubes.
8. Postcoital or Sims-Huhner test (pp. 69–71): microscopic study of a specimen of the female cervical mucus several hours

after intercourse to determine the presence or absence of sperm. At this time, the mucus is also tested for elasticity, and after it has dried on a glass slide, it is examined to determine what it reveals about ovulation (fern test).

9. Vaginal smears (p. 61): microscopic study of vaginal mucus, obtained daily and preserved in a special solution during one menstrual cycle. To determine hormonal changes during the cycle. This test is not always part of the basic evaluation.

Other Tests

10. Hysterosalpingography (pp. 81–82): x-ray study of the uterus and fallopian tubes to determine any abnormality of the uterus or tubes and to test for patency of the tubes. The uterus and tubes are infused with radiopaque dye to make them visible by x-ray.

11. Further hormonal studies (p. 82): laboratory studies in which steroids and gonadotropins are studied extremely closely for hormonal changes. Some of the tests are performed on urine collected during a twenty-four-hour period. Warranted in only 5 to 10 percent of cases of suspected ovulatory dysfunction.

12. Immunologic testing (pp. 82–83): laboratory test of a woman's blood and a man's sperm to determine if there is any immunologic incompatibility.

13. Culdoscopy, laparoscopy, or laparotomy (pp. 83–84): direct examination of the woman's pelvic organs, by opening the pelvic cavity in laparotomy and by using telescopelike devices in culdoscopy or laparoscopy. To determine any abnormalities of uterus, fallopian tubes, or ovaries and to diagnose any other pelvic diseases.

APPENDIX 2

Evaluation of the Man

Basic Preliminary Workup

1. Detailed medical history and physical examination (pp. 73–74.
2. Sexual history (p. 74).
3. Laboratory studies of blood, urine, and thyroid function (p. 74).
4. Analysis of sperm (pp. 74–77): examination of a specimen of sperm to determine the number of milliliters per specimen; the number of sperm per milliliter; the percentage of sperm that are moving (motility); the percentage of sperm that have a normal shape and size (morphology).

One Additional Test

5. Testicular biopsy (p. 84): minor surgical procedure in which a small piece of the testis is removed, treated chemically, and examined under a microscope to determine if spermatogenesis is taking place. Warranted only in certain cases.

APPENDIX 3

Some Organizations Concerned with Infertility

American Fertility Society
1608 Thirteenth Avenue South
Birmingham, Alabama 35205

The Barren Foundation
6 East Monroe Street
Chicago, Illinois 60603

Planned Parenthood of New York City, Inc.
Family Planning and Information Service
300 Park Avenue South
New York, New York 10010

Planned Parenthood — World Population
810 Seventh Avenue
New York, New York 10019

Resolve, Inc.
P.O. Box 474
Belmont, Massachusetts 02178

United Infertility Organization
P.O. Box 23
Scarsdale, New York 10583

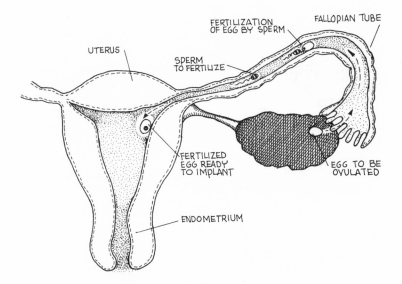

Fig. 1. Diagram of Conception

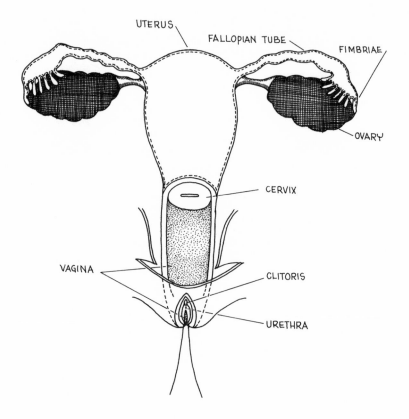

Fig. 2. FEMALE GENITAL ORGANS

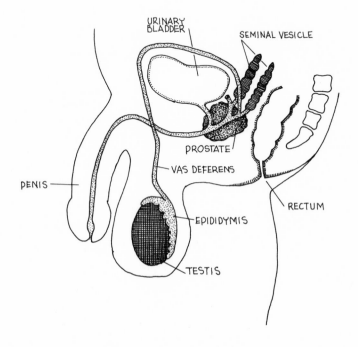

Fig. 3. MALE GENITAL ORGANS

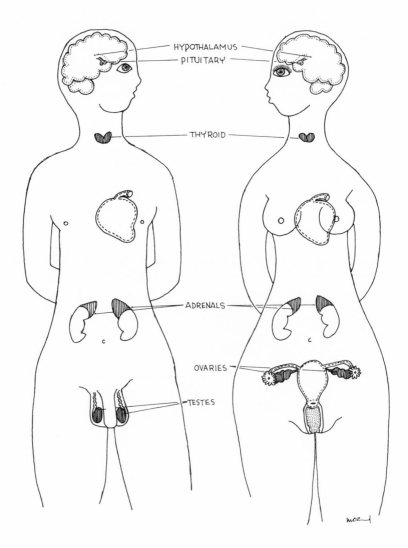

Fig. 4. Glands Involved in Reproduction in the Male and in the Female

MONTH AND DATE

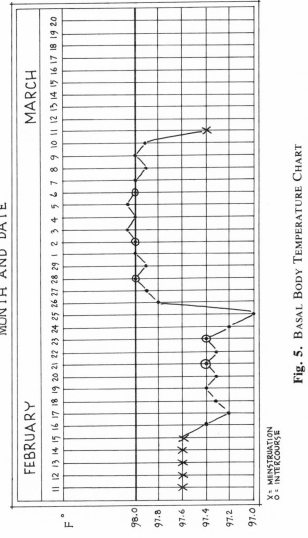

Fig. 5. Basal Body Temperature Chart

The chart shows presumptive evidence of ovulation sometime between February 23 and 27, that is, between days 13 and 17 in the cycle.

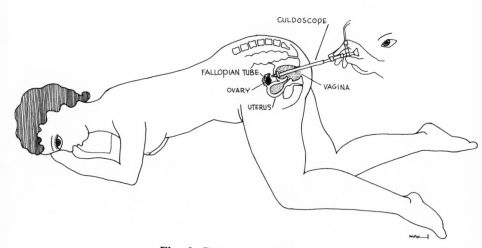

Fig. 6. POSITION FOR CULDOSCOPY

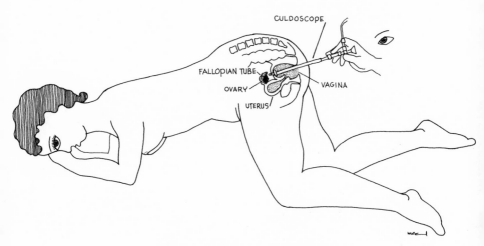

Fig. 6. POSITION FOR CULDOSCOPY

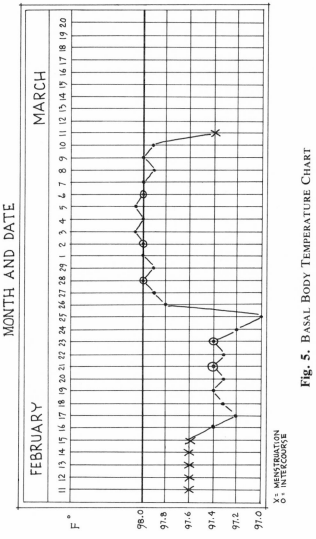

Fig. 5. BASAL BODY TEMPERATURE CHART

The chart shows presumptive evidence of ovulation sometime between February 23 and 27, that is, between days 13 and 17 in the cycle.

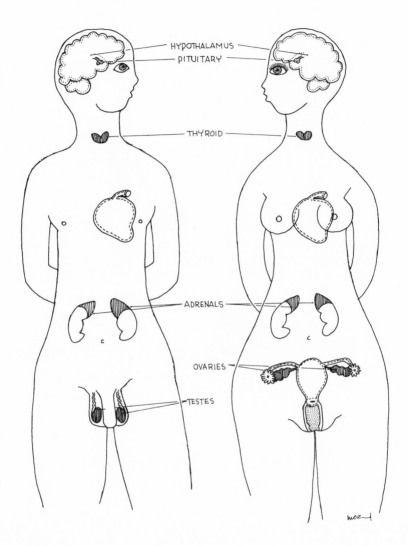

Fig. 4. GLANDS INVOLVED IN REPRODUCTION IN THE MALE AND IN THE FEMALE

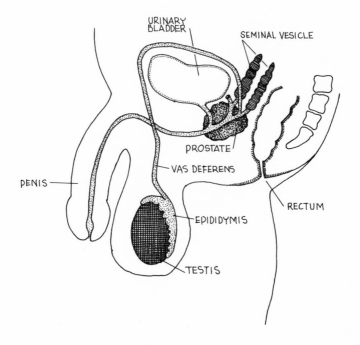

Fig. 3. MALE GENITAL ORGANS

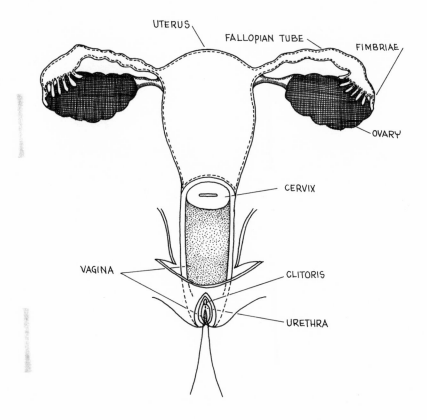

Fig. 2. FEMALE GENITAL ORGANS

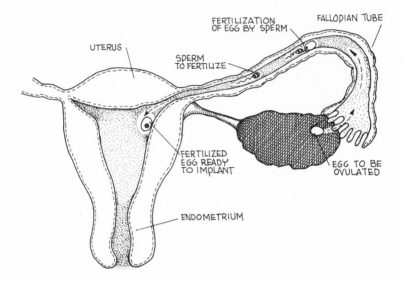

Fig. 1. DIAGRAM OF CONCEPTION

Notes

Chapter 1 (pp. 9–13)

1. Sophia J. Kleegman and Sherwin A. Kaufman, *Infertility in Women* (Philadelphia: F. A. Davis, 1966), p. 4.
2. Ibid.
3. Samuel J. Behrman and Robert W. Kistner, "A Rational Approach to the Evaluation of Infertility," in *Progress in Infertility*, ed. Behrman and Kistner (Boston: Little, Brown, 1968), p. 1, cite a male factor in 30 to 35 percent of all cases, a female factor in 65 to 70 percent; Robert H. Glass and Nathan G. Kase, *Women's Choice* (New York: Basic Books, 1970), p. 67, cite a male factor in 40 percent of cases and a female factor in 60 percent.
4. Behrman and Kistner, "A Rational Approach," pp. 5f., find this in 35 percent of cases; Kleegman and Kaufman, *Infertility in Women*, p. 6, find it in 80 percent of cases.
5. Christopher Tietze, "Reproductive Span and Rate of Reproduction among Hutterite Women," *Fertility and Sterility* 8 (1957): 89–97.
6. Kleegman and Kaufman, *Infertility in Women*, p. 308.

Chapter 2 (pp. 14–20)

1. J. E. Davis, "Clinical Aspects of Male Infertility," in Maxwell Roland, *Management of the Infertile Couple* (Springfield, Illinois: C. C. Thomas, 1968), pp. 67–88.

2. Glass and Kase, *Women's Choice,* p. 12.
3. J. B. Doyle, "Tubo-ovarian mechanism: observation at laparotomy," *Obstetrics and Gynecology* 8 (1956): 686.
4. Ibid.

Chapter 3 (pp. 21–28)

1. Behrman and Kistner, "A Rational Approach," p. 4., cite 5 to 10 percent; Glass and Kase, *Women's Choice,* p. 67, cite 20 percent.
2. Leon Speroff, Robert H. Glass, and Nathan G. Kase, *Clinical Gynecological Endocrinology and Infertility* (Baltimore: Williams and Wilkins, 1973), pp. 206–7.
3. Behrman and Kistner, "A Rational Approach," p. 1; Glass and Kase, *Women's Choice,* p. 67.
4. Carl Tupper and Robert J. Weil, "The Etiology of Habitual Abortion," in *Progress in Infertility,* pp. 751–66.
5. Ibid.

Chapter 4 (pp. 31–36)

1. Behrman and Kistner, "A Rational Approach," p. 2; Anna L. Southam, "What to do with the 'normal' infertile couple?" *Fertility and Sterility* 11 (1960): 543–47.
2. C. Lee Buxton and Anna L. Southam, *Human Infertility* (New York: Hoeber-Harper, 1958), p. 209.
3. Tietze, "Reproductive Span," pp. 89.
4. Melvin Taymor, *The Management of Infertility* (Springfield, Illinois: C. C. Thomas, 1969), p. 9.
5. See Peter Beaconsfield et al., "Amenorrhea and infertility after the use of oral contraceptives," *Surgery, Gynecology, and Obstetrics* 138 (1974): 571–75.
6. Speroff, Glass, and Kase, *Gynecological Endocrinology,* p. 166.
7. Ibid. See also, R. P. Shearman, "Prolonged secondary amenorrhea after oral contraception therapy," *Lancet* 2, no. 7715 (1971): pp. 64ff.

Chapter 5 (pp. 37–46)

1. Taymor, *Management of Infertility,* pp. 5–7.
2. Behrman and Kistner, "A Rational Approach," pp. 5–6.

3. American Fertility Society, eds., *How to Organize a Basic Study of the Infertile Couple,* Birmingham, Alabama, 1971; Planned Parenthood—World Population, *Guide for Couples Seeking Parenthood,* rev. ed., New York, 1975. The Barren Foundation, brochures entitled: *What Does an Infertile Couple Do?; What is Infertility?; Treatment of an Infertile Couple; Artificial Insemination; Psychological Aspects of Fertility; Physiology of Infertility; Female Surgery;* and *Passport to Parenthood.*

Chapter 6 (pp. 47–49)

1 Kleegman and Kaufman, *Infertility in Women,* p. 312.

Chapter 7 (pp. 54–61)

1. Kleegman and Kaufman, *Infertility in Women,* p. 136.
2. C. Lee Buxton and Earl T. Engle, "Time of ovulation: correlation between basal temperature, appearance of endometrium, and appearance of ovary," *American Journal of Obstetrics and Gynecology* 60 (1950): 539–51.
3. Speroff, Glass, and Kase, *Gynecological Endocrinology,* p. 182.
4. Kleegman and Kaufman, *Infertility in Women,* p. 58.
5. Ibid., pp. 36–40.

Chapter 8 (pp. 62–71)

1. Buxton and Southam, *Human Infertility,* p. 156.
2. Speroff, Glass, and Kase, *Gynecological Endocrinology,* p. 177–78.
3. Cyril C. Marcus and Stewart L. Marcus, "The Cervical Factor," in *Progress in Infertility,* p. 41.
4. Ibid., pp. 41–62.

Chapter 9 (pp. 72–78)

1. Matthew Freund, "Semen Analysis," in *Progress in Infertility,* p. 600.
2. John MacLeod, "Seminal cytology in the presence of varicocele," *Fertility and Sterility* 16 (1965): 735.

3. John MacLeod, "Human Male Infertility," *Obstetrical and Gynecological Survey* 26 (1971): 335–36 and 343.
4. Ibid., p. 348.

Chapter 10 (pp. 79–85)

1. Speroff, Glass, and Kase, *Gynecological Endocrinology*, p. 173.
2. Taymor, *Management of Infertility*, p. 60.
3. Bengt Fredricsson, "Laparoscopy versus culdoscopy in the investigation of infertility," *Acta Obstetricia et Gynecologica Scandinavica* 53 (1974): 125. Also Maxwell Roland, "Culdoscopy and laparoscopy: Competitive or complementary technics?" *Fertility and Sterility* 21 (1970): 361–76.
4. E. P. Peterson and S. J. Behrman, "Laparoscopy and Hysteroscopy," *Progress in Infertility*, ed. Behrman and Kistner, 2d ed. rev. (Boston: Little, Brown, 1975), pp. 865–90.
5. Taymor, *Management of Infertility*, pp. 83–84.
6. Buxton and Southam, *Human Infertility*, p. 208.
7. Taymor, *Management of Infertility*, p. 122.

Part Four (pp. 93–95)

1. Kleegman and Kaufman, *Infertility in Women*, p. 261.
2. Speroff, Glass, and Kase, *Gynecological Endocrinology*, pp. 214–22.

Chapter 12 (pp. 96–109)

1. Marcus and Marcus, "The Cervical Factor," p. 56.
2. Taymor, *Management of Infertility*, p. 86.
3. Marcus and Marcus, "The Cervical Factor," p. 58.
4. Kleegman and Kaufman, *Infertility in Women*, pp. 150–52.
5. Ibid.
6. Lawrence J. Malone and Francis M. Ingersoll, "Myomectomy in Infertility," in *Progress in Infertility*, p. 120.
7. Dean L. Moyer, "Endometrial Diseases in Infertility," in *Progress in Infertility*, pp. 128–29.
8. Kleegman and Kaufman, *Infertility in Women*, pp. 54–55.

9. Celso-Ramon Garcia, "Surgical Reconstruction of the Oviduct in the Infertile Patient," in *Progress in Infertility*, p. 256.

10. Taymor, *Management of Infertility*, p. 92.

11. Ibid.

12. Cyril C. Marcus and Stewart L. Marcus, "Advances in Infertility," *Advances in Obstetrics and Gynecology* 1 (1967): 454.

13. Ibid. and Taymor, *Management of Infertility*, p. 101.

14. Garcia, "Surgical Reconstruction," pp. 260–62.

15. Speroff, Glass, and Kase, *Gynecological Endocrinology*, pp. 191–92.

16. Taymor, *Management of Infertility*, p. 101.

17. Joseph W. Goldzieher, "Polycystic Ovarian Disease," in *Progress in Infertility*, p. 371.

18. Richard H. Schwarz, "Acute Pelvic Inflammatory Disease," in *Infectious Diseases in Obstetrics and Gynecology*, ed. Gilles R. G. Monif (New York: Harper and Row, 1974), p. 381.

19. Ibid., p. 384.

20. Samuel Rozin, "Genital Tuberculosis," in *Progress in Infertility*, pp. 209–10.

21. For a summary of opinions, see: Robert W. Kistner, "Endometriosis and Infertility," in *Progress in Infertility*, pp. 327–50. Also J. H. Ridley, "The histogenesis of endometriosis. A review of facts and fancies," *Obstetrical and Gynecological Survey*, 23 (1968): 1–35.

22. Speroff, Glass, and Kase, *Gynecological Endocrinology*, p. 202.

23. Kistner, "Endometriosis," p. 329.

24. Ibid., p. 348.

25. See Speroff, Glass, and Kase, *Gynecological Endocrinology*, pp. 214–22, for a comprehensive account of this kind of therapy.

26. Ibid., p. 220.

27. Ibid.

28. Ibid., p. 222.

29. Ibid.

30. See "Part VIII. Immunological Factors," *Progress in Infertility*, 2d ed. rev., pp. 793–863.

31. Southam, "What to do with the 'normal' infertile couple?" *Fertility and Sterility* 11 (1960): 546–47.

Chapter 14 (pp. 119–126)

1. MacLeod, "Human Male Infertility," *Obstetrical and Gynecological Survey,* 26 (1971): p. 348.
2. Bruce H. Stewart, "Drugs that cause and cure male infertility," *Drug Therapy,* December 1975, p. 49.
3. Taymor, *Management of Infertility,* p. 81.
4. Ibid., p. 82.
5. Stewart, "Drugs," p. 48.
6. Speroff, Glass, and Kase, *Gynecological Endocrinology,* pp. 207–9.
7. Stewart, "Drugs," p. 48.
8. Taymor, *Management of Infertility,* p. 81.
9. Stewart, "Drugs," p. 49.
10. Speroff, Glass, and Kase, *Gynecological Endocrinology,* p. 208.
11. Stewart, "Drugs," p. 49.
12. Ibid.
13. Richard Amelar, *Infertility in Men* (Philadelphia: F. A. Davis, 1966), passim.
14. Tien S. Li, "Sperm immunology, infertility, and fertility control," *Obstetrics and Gynecology* 44 (1974): 611–12.
15. Taymor, *Management of Infertility,* p. 87.
16. Stewart, "Drugs," p. 48.
17. Richard Amelar, "A new method for promoting fertility," *Obstetrics and Gynecology* 45 (1975): 56–59.
18. Y. Sawada and D. R. Ackerman, "Use of Frozen Human Semen," in *Progress in Infertility,* pp. 731–50.
19. Speroff, Glass, and Kase, *Gynecological Endocrinology,* p. 209.
20. Samuel J. Behrman, "Techniques of Artificial Insemination," in *Progress in Infertility,* p. 728.

Chapter 15 (pp. 129–131)

1. Kleegman and Kaufman, *Infertility in Women,* p. 4.
2. Tietze, "Reproductive Span," *Fertility and Sterility* 8 (1957): 89–97.
3. Kleegman and Kaufman, *Infertility in Women,* pp. 327–28.

Chapter 16 (pp. 132–137)

1. Carl Tupper and Robert J. Weil, "The Etiology of Habitual Abortion," *Progress in Infertility,* p. 752.
2. Kleegman and Kaufman, *Infertility in Women,* p. 225.
3. Ibid., p. 224.
4. Tupper and Weil, "Etiology of Habitual Abortion," pp. 751–65 for a review of theories.
5. Kleegman and Kaufman, p. 224.
6. Tupper and Weil, "Etiology of Habitual Abortion," p. 755.
7. Ibid., p. 762. See also W. R. Jones and S. J. Behrman, "Immunological Aspects of Placentation," *Progress in Infertility,* 2d ed. rev., pp. 817–44.
8. Tupper and Weil, pp. 755–56.

Chapter 17 (pp. 138–141)

1. These include: local community, family, and children's service agencies; community council or welfare planning bodies; and state welfare departments. On the national level, contact: the Child Welfare League of America, 67 Irving Place, New York City, or the Office of Child Development, Children's Bureau, Department of Health, Education, and Welfare, Washington, D.C.
2. John Rock, Christopher Tietze, Helen B. McLaughlin, "Effect of Adoption on Infertility," *Fertility and Sterility* 16 (1965): 305–12. Also William C. Weir and David R. Weir, "Adoption and Subsequent Conceptions," *Fertility and Sterility* 17 (1966): 283.
3. Rock, Tietze, and McLaughlin, "Effect of Adoption," p. 312.
4. Sherwin A. Kaufman, *New Hope for the Childless Couple,* (New York: Simon and Schuster, 1970), pp. 119–20.

Chapter 18 (pp. 147–152)

1. Speroff, Glass, and Kase, *Gynecological Endocrinology,* p. 166.
2. Ibid.
3. Celso-Ramon Garcia and Amnon David, "Longterm effects of oral contraceptives on ovary and pituitary," *International Journal of Fertility* 13 (1968): 292.

4. William C. Andrews, "Oral contraception: A review of reported physiological and pathological effects," *Obstetrical and Gynecological Survey* 26 (1971): 492.

5. Hugh J. Davis, *Intrauterine Devices for Contraception* (Baltimore: Williams and Wilkins, 1971), p. 109.

6. S. D. Targum and N. H. Wright, "Association of IUD and PID: a retrospective pilot study," *American Journal of Epidemiology* 100 (1974): 262–71. See also: L. R. Weekes, "Complications of the intrauterine contraceptive device," *Journal of the National Medical Association* 67 (1975): 1–10.

7. Davis, *Intrauterine Devices*, p. 107.

8. Weekes, "Complications of intrauterine device," pp. 7–8.

9. Ibid.

10. Ibid.

11. Jane E. Brody, "Microsurgery Successful in Vasectomy Reversals," in *New York Times*, 8 October 1975.

12. Tien S. Li, "Sperm immunology, infertility, and fertility control," *Obstetrics and Gynecology* 44 (1974): 611–12.

13. Alan Guttmacher, *Babies by Choice or by Chance* (New York: Avon Book Division, 1961), p. 70.

14. Philip D. Harvey, "Condoms, a new look," *Family Planning Perspectives* 4 no. 22 (1972): 29.

15. Andrews, "Oral Contraception," p. 487.

Chapter 20 (pp. 158–160)

1. Jane E. Brody, "Microsurgery Successful in Vasectomy Reversals," in *New York Times,* 8 October 1975.

2. Samuel J. Behrman, "Preservation of Human Sperm by Nitrogen Vapor Freezing," *Current Problems in Fertility,* ed. A. Ingelman-Sundberg and N.-O. Lunell (New York: Plenum Press, 1971), pp. 10–16. See also: Y. Sawada and D. R. Ackerman, "Use of Frozen Human Semen," *Progress in Infertility,* pp. 731–50.

3. Max Amoss and Roger Guillemin, "Hypothalamus and Anterior Pituitary," *Progress in Infertility,* 2d ed. rev., pp. 539–62.

4. M. Kirimura, J. Ono, and M. Hayashi, "The Experimental Artificial Oviduct," *Current Problems in Fertility,* pp. 229–30.

5. S. Kullander, "Medical Aspects of Transplants in Gynecology," *Current Problems in Fertility,* pp. 62–65.

6. P. Vara, M. Seppälä, and S. Paatsma, "Significance of Transplantation of the Uterus and Fallopian Tubes," *Current Problems in Fertility,* pp. 81–83.

7. L. Gedda, "Transplantation of Gynecological Organs: Ethical Problems," *Current Problems in Fertility,* pp. 57–61, and "In vitro fertilization of human ova and blastocyst transfer. An invitational symposium," *Journal of Reproductive Medicine* 2 (1973): 192–200.

8. R. G. Edwards and P. C. Steptoe, "Physiological Aspects of Human Embryo Transfer," *Progress in Infertility,* 2d ed. rev., pp. 377–410.

Selected Bibliography

Medical Books and Articles of Interest to Laymen

FOR SPECIFIC topics, readers are urged to consult works cited in the Notes.

Amelar, Richard. *Infertility in Men.* Philadelphia: F. A. Davis, 1966. A comprehensive text on male infertility.

Behrman, Samuel J., and Robert W. Kistner. "A Rational Approach to the Evaluation of Infertility." *Progress in Infertility.* Edited by Behrman and Kistner. Boston: Little Brown, 1968. 1–20. A short and sensible summation of current thinking about the evaluation of infertility.

Behrman, Samuel J., and Robert W. Kistner, eds. *Progress in Infertility.* Boston: Little Brown, 1968. A comprehensive collection of articles on various aspects of infertility by experts in each field. The Second Edition, Revised, appeared too late to be consulted extensively. However, I have mentioned in footnotes some articles in the second edition with new or updated material.

Buxton, C. Lee, and Anna L. Southam. *Human Infertility.* New York: Hoeber-Harper, 1958. A textbook that is very sensitive to the complexities of the study of infertility as well as to the suffering of patients.

Kleegman, Sophia J., and Sherwin A. Kaufman. *Infertility in Women.* Philadelphia: F. A. Davis, 1966. A textbook that humanely keeps in mind the needs of patients while presenting a very thorough method for evaluating infertility. Case histories are included.

MacLeod, John. "Human Male Infertility." *Obstetrical and Gynecological Survey* 26 (1971): 335–51. A comprehensive review of current thinking on male infertility by one of the leading experts in the field.

Speroff, Leon, Robert H. Glass, and Nathan C. Kase. *Clinical Gynecological Endocrinology and Infertility*. Baltimore: Williams and Wilkins, 1973. A textbook for physicians on the complex field of gynecological endocrinology. The section on infertility surveys the problem and gives an especially thorough picture of endocrinological problems and their treatment.

Roland, Maxwell. *Management of the Infertile Couple*. Springfield, Illinois: C. C. Thomas, 1968. A textbook on infertility with articles on male problems by experts in the field.

Taymor, Melvin. *The Management of Infertility*. Springfield, Illinois: C. C. Thomas, 1969. A textbook written by an expert for nonspecialist physicians. A concise survey of the field with special attention to possible pitfalls as well as to the needs of patients.

Glossary of Medical Terms

Adrenal glands: two small glands near the kidneys that produce adrenalin, cortisone, and small amounts of some sexual hormones

Adrenogenital syndrome: syndrome caused by an overactivity of the adrenal glands, resulting in the appearance of secondary male sexual characteristics in the female

Agglutination of sperm: the clumping together of sperm

Amniocentesis: procedure in which a small amount of amniotic fluid is removed from the uterus of a pregnant woman to examine it for the presence of abnormal cells of the fetus

Androgen: generic name for male sexual hormones

Anovulation: the cessation or suspension of ovulation

Appendicitis: inflammation of the appendix, usually caused by infection

Artificial insemination: see Donor therapeutic insemination and Husband therapeutic insemination

Azoospermia: lack of sperm in the semen

Basal Body Temperature Chart (BBT): chart of a female's body temperature taken daily throughout a menstrual cycle. Can provide presumptive evidence of the presence or absence of ovulation.

Bicornuate uterus: congenital malformation of the uterus in which the upper part is divided into two hornlike projections

Blastocyst: the fertilized egg during its earliest stages of development

Caesarean section: surgical delivery of a baby through incisions cut in the mother's abdomen and uterus

Cannula: hollow tube

Cervical polyps: benign growths on the cervix

Cervix: lower part or neck of the uterus which protrudes in the vaginal canal and which contains an opening (os cervix) leading into the uterus

Cilia: minuscule hairlike forms inside the fallopian tubes. Their undulant motion apparently helps to push the egg toward the uterus.

Clomid: brand name of clomiphene citrate, a synthetic drug that attempts to stimulate the functioning of the pituitary gland

Coitus interruptus: intercourse in which the male withdraws his penis from the vagina before ejaculation

Condom: male contraceptive device that covers the penis during intercourse

Congenital: existing at birth

Conization: surgical procedure in which infected or inflamed parts of the cervix are excised

Contraception: the artificial prevention of conception, also known as birth control

Corpus luteum (Latin for "yellow body"): yellow mass in the ovary, formed from a follicle that has produced and released an egg. The corpus luteum is apparently responsible for the secretion of progesterone.

Cortisone: hormone produced by the adrenal glands with many functions relating to many systems of the body

Culdoscopy: minor surgical procedure in which a telescopelike device is inserted into the female abdominal cavity through a slit in the vagina near the cervix. This procedure allows visual examination of the female pelvic organs.

Cytomel: a thyroid medication

Diaphragm: female contraceptive device that covers the cervix and prevents sperm from entering the uterus.

Donor therapeutic insemination (also known as donor artificial insemination or A.I.D.): medical procedure in which the semen from an unknown donor is placed by a physician in the vagina of a woman. See also Husband therapeutic insemination.

Dyspareunia: pain on intercourse

Ectopic pregnancy: pregnancy that implants outside the uterus

Electrocauterization: procedure in which infected or inflamed parts of the cervix are burned off with an electrical instrument

Embryo: developing stage of a fertilized egg from one week after conception to the end of the second month

Endocrine system: system of glands in men and women including the thymus, pituitary, thyroid, adrenals, testicles or ovaries.

Endometrial adhesions: fibrous adhesions in the lining of the uterus

Endometrial biopsy: minor surgical procedure in which a small piece of the endometrium is removed in order to examine it under a microscope

Endometriosis: condition in which endometrial-like tissue is present outside the uterus

Endometrium: mucous membrane lining the cavity of the uterus

Epididymis: oblong structure attached to each testicle where sperm collect on their way to the vas deferens

Estrogen: female sexual hormone produced primarily by the ovary in women and, in very small amounts, by the adrenal glands in both men and women

Fallopian tubes: two tubes, extending from the upper part of the uterus into the abdominal cavity, through which the egg passes from the ovary to the uterus

Fern test: study of dried cervical mucus that can provide presumptive evidence of ovulation

Fetus: human developing in the uterus from the end of the second month; known as embryo prior to that stage

Fibroid tumor: benign fibrous growth, usually in the muscular structure of the uterus

Fimbriae: fringelike outer end of the fallopian tubes

Fimbriolysis: surgical procedure in which the fimbriae of the fallopian tubes are freed from adhesions

Follicle: egg sac in the ovary

Follicle-stimulating hormone (FSH): hormone put out by the pituitary gland that stimulates the growth of egg follicles in the female ovary and spermatogenesis in the male testicle

Frigidity: sexual indifference or aversion or failure to experience sexual arousal; term usually applied to the female

FSH: see above

Gland: any hormone-producing organ of the body

Gonadotropin: substance capable of stimulating the testicles or ovaries

Gonorrhea: contagious inflammation of the genital tract, caused by the gonococcus bacteria and transmitted chiefly through intercourse

Gynecologist: physician specializing in reproductive physiology and diseases of women

HCG or human chorionic gonadotropin: substance extracted from the urine of pregnant women that can be administered by injection to stimulate the gonads, ovaries, or testicles

HMG or human menopausal gonadotropin: see Pergonal

Hormone: secretion from any of the endocrine glands

Husband therapeutic insemination (also known as husband artificial insemination or A.I.H.): medical procedure in which the husband's semen is placed by a physician in the wife's vagina

Hymen: membrane at the opening of the vagina that partially or fully blocks it

Hypospadias: malformation of the penis in which the opening is located on the underside of the head of the penis.

Hypothalamus: region of the brain situated above the pituitary gland and considered by many to be the "master control" of all the glands

Hypothyroidism: deficiency of the thyroid gland that results in an underproduction of thyroid hormones

Hysterectomy: surgical removal of the uterus

Hysterosalpingography: x-ray study of the uterus and fallopian tubes, which have been infused with radio-opaque dye to make them visible by x ray

ICSH: see Interstitial cell-stimulating hormone

Immunologic testing: laboratory testing of the compatibility of the male's sperm and the female's blood

Impotence: inability of a male to have an erection of the penis

Interstitial cell: minuscule cells located between the seminiferous tubules in the testicles and involved in the production of testosterone

Interstitial cell-stimulating hormone (ICSH): hormone put out by the pituitary gland in men to stimulate the production of testosterone in the interstitial cells of the testicles. Similar to luteinizing hormone in women.

Intrauterine device (IUD): female contraceptive device that is placed in the uterus by a physician to prevent pregnancy

IUD: see above

Laparoscopy: surgical procedure in which a telescopelike device is inserted into a woman's abdominal cavity through an incision in her abdomen to allow visual examination of the pelvic organs

Laparotomy: surgical procedure to explore the abdominal cavity

Luteal phase: second part of a woman's menstrual cycle, when a mature egg has been released from the ovary and the corpus luteum has been formed and is causing the production of progesterone

Luteinizing hormone (LH): hormone put out by the pituitary gland in women that causes the release of a mature egg from an ovarian follicle. Similar to ICSH in men.

Menopause: cessation of menstruation that accompanies the end of a female's fertility

Menstruation: monthly shedding of the lining of the uterus that occurs in the absence of pregnancy

Morphology of sperm: study of the shape and structure of sperm

Motility of sperm: ability of sperm to propel themselves forward by means of the whiplike motions of their tails

Mumps orchitis: inflammation of the testicle caused by the mumps virus

Myomectomy: surgical excision of fibroid tumors of the uterus, leaving the uterus intact

Ob-gyn: see Obstetrician-gynecologist

Obstetrician-gynecologist: physician specializing in the reproductive physiology of women, in women's diseases, and in the management of pregnancy, labor, and delivery

Oligospermia: deficiency in the number of sperm in the semen

Orchitis: inflammation of the testicle. See Mumps orchitis

Ovary: female sexual gland that produces the eggs and female hormones, located near the uterus and the fallopian tubes

Oviduct: fallopian tube

Ovulation: expulsion of a mature egg from a follicle in the ovary

Ovum (pl. ova): egg or eggs produced in the female ovary

Pap smear: screening test developed by George Papanicolaou to determine malignant cells in the cervical mucus

Pelvic inflammatory disease (also known as PID): general name for inflammatory diseases of the pelvis; can be caused by gonorrhea, peritonitis, tuberculosis, or other infections

Penis: male sexual organ

Pergonal: brand name for an injectable preparation containing human menopausal gonadotropin (HMG), a substance extracted from the urine of menopausal women that is capable of stimulating the gonads, ovaries or testicles

Peritoneal cavity: abdominal cavity

Peritoneum: membrane lining the abdominal cavity

Peritonitis: inflammation of the membrane lining the abdominal cavity

Peritubal adhesions: adhesions of tissue around the fallopian tubes

Pituitary gland: gland located at the base of the brain that affects growth and sexual functioning in both men and women

Polycystic ovaries: formation of multiple cysts in the ovaries, probably representing a failure of the ovaries to discharge eggs

Postcoital test (also known as Sims-Huhner test): study of a sample of the female cervical mucus several hours after intercourse to determine the presence of sperm

Premature ejaculation: ejaculation of sperm from the penis prior to or immediately after entering the vagina

Progesterone: female hormone, produced by the corpus luteum in the ovary, that helps to stimulate the growth of a uterine lining capable of receiving and nourishing a fertilized egg

Prostate gland: gland located near the bladder and urethra in the male that supplies part of the fluid of the semen

Psychosomatic: used to describe physical symptoms caused by or aggravated by psychological or emotional tensions

Puberty: age of sexual maturity

Retrograde ejaculation: condition in men in which sperm are ejaculated into the bladder rather than out through the penis

Retroverted uterus: malpositioned uterus that is flexed severely forward or backward

Rubin test: see Tubal insufflation

Salpingolysis: surgical procedure to free the fallopian tubes from adhesions

Salpingoplasty: surgical procedure to correct blocked fallopian tubes

Scrotum: sac that contains the male testicles and accessory organs

Semen: liquid produced by the male reproductive organs that contains sperm and other secretions

Seminiferous tubules: small tubes in the testicles where sperm are produced

Sims-Huhner test: see Postcoital test

Speculum: instrument that is inserted in the female vagina to allow the visualization of the cervix

Sperm (spermatozoon, pl. spermatozoa): male germ cell, produced in the testicles, consisting of a small head containing the chromosomes, a neck, and a tail

Spermatogenesis: creation of sperm

Spinnbarkeit: elasticity of the cervical mucus

Stein-Leventhal disease: female syndrome that can have symptoms including infertility, polycystic ovaries, excess hair growth on face and body, and occasionally obesity

Steroids: chemical compounds characterized by a similar structure, including cortisone and its derivatives and some sex hormones

Testicle (Latin, *testis*, pl. *testes*): male sexual gland where sperm are produced; located in the scrotum

Testicular biopsy: minor surgical procedure in which a small piece of the testicle is removed to determine if spermatogenesis is taking place

Testis, testes: see Testicle

Testosterone: male sexual hormone produced in the interstitial cells of the testicles and responsible for male sexual characteristics

Thrombophlebitis: formation of blood clots in the veins, usually preceded by inflammation of the vein itself

Thyroid gland: gland located in the neck that produces thyroxin

Thyroxin: hormone produced by the thyroid gland

"Tipped" uterus: see Retroverted uterus

Tubal insufflation (Rubin test): test in which carbon dioxide is passed through the uterus and fallopian tubes to determine if the fallopian tubes are open

Tubal patency: condition in which the fallopian tubes are unobstructed and open

Urethra: canal to carry urine from the bladder to outside of the body. In the male it also carries the seminal ejaculation.

Urologist: physician specializing in the physiology and diseases of the genitourinary tract in men and women and in infertility in men

Uterine suspension: surgical procedure in which the uterus is sutured to the abdominal wall

Uterus: female reproductive organ, a hollow muscular structure in which the embryo and fetus grow

Vagina: canal between the vulva and the cervix in the woman into which the male inserts his penis during intercourse. The opening of the vagina is located in the vulva between the urethra and the rectum.

Vaginismus: extreme constriction of the vagina which prevents intercourse or makes it extremely difficult

Varicocele: dilation of the testicular veins of the spermatic cord

Varicocelectomy: surgical procedure to remove dilated testicular veins

Vas deferens (pl., vasa deferentia): passage that carries sperm from the testicle to the ejaculatory duct

Vasectomy: surgical procedure in which the vas deferens, or a part of it, is excised

Wedge resection: surgical procedure in which a small section is cut out of the ovary and the ovary is resutured

Index